MANAGEMENT OF OSTEOARTHRITIS OF THE KNEE:

AN INTERNATIONAL CONSENSUS

EDITED BY
FREDDIE H. FU, MD
UNIVERSITY OF PITTSBURGH SCHOOL OF MEDICINE
PITTSBURGH, PENNSYLVANIA

BRUCE D. BROWNER, MD
UCONN HEALTH CENTER
FARMINGTON, CONNECTICUT

American Academy of Orthopaedic Surgeons

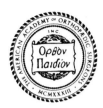

American Academy of Orthopaedic Surgeons
6300 North River Road
Rosemont, IL 60018
1-800-626-6726

The American Academy of Orthopaedic Surgeons Monograph Series is dedicated to Wendy O. Schmidt, American Academy of Orthopaedic Surgeons senior medical editor from 1987 to 1991.

First Edition
Copyright © 2003 by the
American Academy of Orthopaedic Surgeons

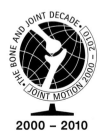

2000 – 2010

CONTRIBUTORS

Rene Jorge Abdala, MD
Orthopaedic Department
Federal University of Sao Paulo
Sao Paulo, Brazil

Frederick Almquist, MD, PhD
Orthopaedic Surgeon
Department of Orthopaedic Surgery
Ghent University Hospital
Ghent, Belgium

Joicemar T. Amaro, MD
Orthopaedic Department
Federal University of Sao Paulo
Sao Paulo, Brazil

Philippe Cartier, MD
Knee Department
Les Lilas Medical Center
Les Lilas, France

Guglielmo Cerullo, MD
Orthopaedic Surgeon
Clinica Valle Giulia
Private Hospital
Rome, Italy

Massimo Cipolla, MD
Specialist in Orthopaedics
Specialist in Sports Medicine
Sports Traumatology
Clinical Valle Giulia
Rome, Italy

Moisés Cohen, MD
Orthopaedic Department
Federal University of Sao Paulo
Sao Paulo, Brazil

Benno Ejnisman, MD
Orthopaedic Department
Federal University of Sao Paulo
Sao Paulo, Brazil

Vittorio Franco, MD
Orthopaedic Surgeon
Clinica Valle Giulia
Private Hospital
Rome, Italy

Enrico Gianni, MD
Orthopaedic Surgeon
Clinica Valle Giulia
Private Hospital
Rome, Italy

László Hangody, MD, PhD, DSc
Head of the Department
Orthopaedic and Trauma Department
Uzsoki Hospital
Budapest, Hungary

Jodi F. Hartman, MS
Orthopaedic Research & Reporting, Ltd.
Gahanna, Ohio

Elizaveta Kon, MD
Biomechanics Laboratory
Rizzoli Orthopaedic Institute
Bologna, Italy

Masahiro Kurosaka, MD
Professor and Chairman
Department of Orthopaedic Surgery
Kobe University Graduate School of Medicine
Kobe, Japan

Maurilio Marcacci, MD
Biomechanics Laboratory
Rizzoli Orthopaedic Institute
Bologna, Italy

Hirotsugu Muratsu, MD
Assistant Professor
Department of Orthopaedic Surgery
Kobe University Graduate School of Medicine
Kobe, Japan

CONTRIBUTORS (CONT.)

Giancarlo Puddu, MD
Orthopaedic Surgeon
Clinica Valle Giulia
Private Hospital
Rome, Italy

Gábor K. Ráthonyi, MD
Orthopaedic Surgeon
Orthopaedic and Trauma Department
Uzsoki Hospital
Budapest, Hungary

John A. Repicci, MD
Joint Reconstruction Orthopedic Center
Buffalo, New York

René Verdonk, MD, PhD
Professor of Orthopaedic Surgery
Department of Orthopaedic Surgery
Ghent University Hospital
Ghent, Belgium

Alberto Vascellari, MD
Biomechanics Laboratory
Rizzoli Orthopaedic Institute
Bologna, Italy

Molly T. Vogt, PhD
Associate Professor of Orthopaedic
Surgery and Epidemiology
Orthopaedic Surgery Department
University of Pittsburgh
Pittsburgh, Pennsylvania

Shinichi Yoshiya, MD
Associate Professor
Department of Orthopaedic Surgery
Kobe University Graduate School of Medicine
Kobe, Japan

Stefano Zaffagnini, MD
Biomechanics Laboratory
Rizzoli Orthopaedic Institute
Bologna, Italy

CONTENTS

PREFACE

Designed to provide a new avenue of communication for the international orthopaedic community to share important information with the audience at the Annual Meeting of the American Academy of Orthopaedic Surgeons, the International Symposium was initiated at the Dallas meeting in 2002. A controversial and challenging problem for many orthopaedic surgeons—the management of degenerative knee arthritis in the active middle-aged patient—was chosen as the topic of the first symposium. As significant treatments had been developed outside North America, and international surgeons had extensive experience with some techniques, this symposium provided an opportunity for teaching by true experts.

The presentations by this extraordinary panel drawn from Europe, South America, and Asia were so outstanding that we felt they could serve as the basis for a monograph on the same topic. Additional authors from North America were added to fill in the uncovered topics and transform the written symposium into a more collaborative international endeavor. As osteoarthritis is a major focus of the Bone and Joint Decade, the choice of this subject for the first AAOS International Symposium and a subsequent monograph had even more impetus.

We are indebted to our authors for sharing their experience on the subject. Readers will benefit from the clear explanations of each technique and the careful discussion of outcomes. Management of degenerative arthritis of the knee in the active adult is a major challenge. Most of these patients are too young and active to be good candidates for total joint replacement, making it necessary to rely on other treatments. The chapters in this monograph include the thoughts of acknowledged leaders in this field.

We would like to express our gratitude to the Academy staff that made this project possible. In her role as managing editor, Lynne Shindoll communicated with the authors to obtain the various contributions and assemble the manuscript. Joan Abern, Senior Editor, refined the original manuscripts to produce a monograph that "speaks" with one voice. We appreciate their efforts and those of everyone in the Publications Department who consistently produce excellent materials for orthopaedists.

Freddie H. Fu, MD
Bruce D. Browner, MD

CHAPTER *1*

EPIDEMIOLOGY OF KNEE OSTEOARTHRITIS

MOLLY T. VOGT, PHD

Osteoarthritis (OA) is the most common form of arthritis and is a leading cause of disability in older adults in Europe, Canada, Australia, the United Kingdom, and the United States. According to the World Health Organization, about 40 million people in the United States currently have arthritis, and that number is predicted to increase to 60 million by 2020. The economic and social costs of OA are substantial. On average, a person with OA makes nine visits to a physician each year and has 0.2 to 0.3 hospitalizations each year lasting 7 to 8 days each. Functional limitations are reported by about 20% of community dwelling people with OA. Among people aged 51 to 61 years with arthritis, 40% report work-related disability. In 1996, the total costs in the United States for arthritis care were estimated to represent 2.4% of the gross national product or $125 billion; $82 billion is attributed to indirect costs resulting from lost productivity and $43 billion to direct medical costs. The proportion of expenditures for direct costs is rising, in part because of the increased use of joint surgery and increased costs for the new drugs available for treatment.[1]

DEFINITION OF DISEASE

The current definition of osteoarthritis was developed at a conference sponsored by the American Academy of Orthopaedic Surgeons and the National Institutes of Health in 1994.[2]

"OA diseases are a result of both mechanical and biologic events that destabilize the normal coupling of degradation and synthesis of articular cartilage chrondrocytes and extracellular matrix, and subchondral bone. ... Ultimately, OA diseases are manifested by morphologic, biochemical, molecular, and biomechanical changes of both cells and matrix which lead to a softening, fibrillation, ulceration, loss of articular cartilage, sclerosis, and eburnation of subchondral bone, osteophytes, and subchondral cysts. ..."

This definition emphasizes that OA is a dynamic disease of the synovial joint with multiple etiologies. The entire joint is involved in the pathogenesis as are the soft tissues around the joint. Joint failure occurs when excessive or abnormal loading of the joint causes the tissues to fail or when the loading is normal but the tissues fail for other reasons, such as genetic abnormalities or trauma. The primary symptoms are joint pain, stiffness, and decreased mobility.[3]

OA in peripheral joints most frequently involves the knee joint, and the disease may affect one or more of the three compartments of the knee (medial tibiofemoral, lateral tibiofemoral, and patellofemoral). The knee joint acts to transfer force from the thigh muscles to the leg to move the body. Loads exerted on the surfaces of the knee joint during normal daily activities are two to seven times the body weight. Osteoarthritic changes in the joint decrease the effectiveness of load transfer during these activities. Overall mobility is impaired, and knee OA has been shown

TABLE 1

Criteria for Classification of Idiopathic OA of the Knee

Clinical and Laboratory*	Clinical and Radiographic	Clinical†
Knee pain plus at least five of nine of the following:	Knee pain plus at least one of three of the following:	Knee pain plus at least one of six of the following:
Age >50 years	Age >50 years	Age >50 years
Stiffness <30 minutes	Stiffness <30 minutes	Stiffness <30 minutes
Crepitus	Crepitus	Crepitus
Bony tenderness	+	Bony tenderness
Bony enlargement	Osteophytes	Bony enlargement
No palpable warmth		No palpable warmth
ESR <40 mm/h		
RF <1:40		
SF OA		
92% sensitive	91% sensitive	95% sensitive
75% specific	86% specific	69% specific

*ESR, erthrocyte sedimentation rate (Westergren); RF, rheumatoid factor; SF OA, synovial fluid signs of OA (clear, viscous, or white blood cell count <2,000/mm^3).
†Alternative for the clinical category would be four of six of the following, which is 84% sensitive and 89% specific.

Reproduced with permission from Altman R, Asch E, Bloch G, et al: Development of criteria for the classification and reporting of osteoarthritis: Classification of osteoarthritis of the knee. *Arthritis Rheum* 1986;29:1039-1049.

to account for more limitations in walking, stair climbing, or other daily activities than any other disease.

The American College of Rheumatology has developed diagnostic criteria for knee OA using either clinical and laboratory findings or clinical, laboratory, and radiographic findings (Table 1). Most epidemiologic studies use only structural radiographic features to categorize the presence or absence of knee OA. The presence of radiographic findings consistent with Kellgren and Lawrence grades 2 to 4,[4] that is, the presence of osteophytes, is the most common epidemiologic definition of knee OA. This definition is problematic because more than 50% of individuals with radiographically defined knee OA do not report joint pain (Table 2). Conversely, persons with clinically defined OA often have no radiographic abnormalities. This means that the patient population treated for OA differs from the population included in most of the large epidemiologic studies to date. In addition, most studies do not consider the differential involvement of each of the three compartments of the knee in the disease process.

A few recent studies have suggested that the risk factors for development of OA may vary by compartment.

PREVALENCE AND INCIDENCE: EFFECT OF AGE, GENDER, AND RACE

The prevalence of knee OA rises sharply with age, and after menopause is higher in women than men (Figure 1). Reported estimates of prevalence vary widely as a result of varying definitions of disease and characteristics of the cohorts studied. White populations in developed countries have similar prevalence rates. In the first National Health and Nutrition Examination Survey (NHANES I),[5] African-American women, but not men, had a higher prevalence of knee OA than whites. However, the Johnson County Arthritis Project in North Carolina[6] found similar prevalence rates in African-American and white cohorts. The prevalence of knee OA is 45% higher in Chi-

TABLE 2

Relationship Between Radiographic Evidence of Knee OA and Percent of Individuals With Knee Pain

Kellgren and Lawrence Grade	% Patients With Pain
0	8
1	11
2	19
3 or 4	40 to 56

FIGURE 1

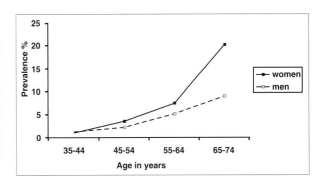

Prevalence of radiographic knee OA in the US population: NHANES I.[5]

FIGURE 2

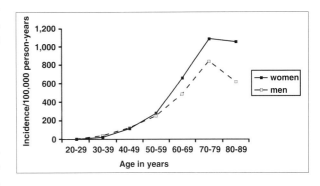

Incidence of knee OA among members of the Fallon Community Health Plan, 1991-1992.[9]

nese women and 100% higher in Japanese women than in white women of a comparable age.[7,8] These ethnic variations may be due to genetic, lifestyle, biologic, or socioeconomic factors.

The incidence of symptomatic OA among patients seeking care in a large health maintenance organization is 2.4 per 1,000 person-years. The incidence increases with age (Figure 2).

RISK FACTORS FOR KNEE OSTEOARTHRITIS

Risk factors for knee OA are usually categorized as systemic factors (age, gender, race, genetic factors, dietary factors, smoking, bone density, estrogen deficiency), which influence susceptibility to the disease, and local factors (obesity, knee alignment, proprioception, laxity, physical activity, periarticular muscle weakness, occupational stress, injury), which affect the distribution of the load across the knee joint (Table 3). However, the etiology of knee OA is influenced by multiple and complex interactions among these factors.[10-12] For example, the aging process usually is accompanied by decreased proprioception and muscle strength, whereas dietary deficiencies may affect cartilage and bone metabolism.

Systemic Risk Factors

Genetic Factors

Genetic factors clearly play a major role in the etiology of generalized OA, but the heritability appears to vary by joint site. Generalized OA appears to be a polygenic condition, and several genome-wide scans are being undertaken to identify the loci that confer susceptibility to OA.[13]

Current evidence indicates that heritability is higher among women than men and may be as high as 60% for

hand and hip OA but is considerably lower for knee OA (estimates range from 10% to 39%). In several epidemiologic studies, the heritability of knee OA was too low for linkage information to be derived, and this has hampered research into the genetics of knee OA.[10,13]

Dietary Factors

Research has suggested that the presence of free oxygen radicals is related to tissue damage in a variety of age-related diseases.[10-12] Chondrocytes are known to reduce free radicals, and it is postulated that these oxidative species may damage the articular cartilage. Antioxidants such as vitamins A, C, and E have the potential to protect against such damage, and data from the Framingham Study[14] support this hypothesis. Subjects in this study were ranked by vitamin C intake, and those in the middle and highest tertiles were found to have a 60% to 70% reduc-

TABLE 3

Risk Factors for Knee OA

Systemic Risk Factors	Local Risk Factors
Age	Obesity
Gender	Joint mechanics (alignment,
Race/ethnicity	proprioception, laxity)
Genetic factors	Muscle weakness
Dietary factors (?)	(quadriceps)
Smoking (?)	Occupational stress
Estrogen deficiency (?)	Physical activity
	Knee injury

tion in risk for progressive knee OA compared with those in the lowest tertile. High vitamin C levels also were associated with a reduced risk for knee pain but appear to have no influence on the development of new cases of radiographic knee OA.

Vitamin D plays an important role in bone mineralization and may influence the response of bone during the arthritic process.[10] Data from the Framingham study indicate that although neither vitamin D intake nor serum levels of 25-hydroxy vitamin D are related to the incidence of knee OA, high levels are protective against progression of disease.[8]

Bone Mineral Density
About 30 years ago surgeons reported that the excised bone from elderly patients with osteoporotic hip fractures rarely showed osteoarthritic changes. Since that time many cross-sectional and case-control studies have confirmed the inverse relationship between osteoporosis and OA.[12,15]

Persons with knee or hip OA usually have 5% to 10% higher bone mineral density (BMD) than those with no OA, regardless of the site at which the BMD is measured. Two recent prospective studies have confirmed that women who developed knee OA during the course of the study had higher BMD (measured at baseline several years earlier) than those who did not develop knee OA.[16,17] BMD was not related to progression of knee OA, defined as an increase in Kellgren and Lawrence grade from 2 (presence of osteophytes) to 3 (joint space narrowing).[4]

There is growing evidence of a relationship between the pathogenesis of OA and bone metabolism. Antiresorptive agents, such as calcitonin and bisphosphonates, have been shown to prevent osteophyte formation and cartilage breakdown in animals. Currently a randomized clinical trial is in progress to determine whether bisphosphonate therapy (risedronate) will influence the progression of knee OA.

Estrogen Deficiency
The incidence of knee OA in women increases sharply after menopause, suggesting that estrogen deficiency may be an etiologic factor.[10,12] The relationship between estrogen replacement therapy (ERT) and knee OA has been considered in several cross-sectional and prospective studies.[18-21] In most, but not all, ERT was found to be associated with a reduced likelihood for OA. A dose-response relationship, that is, that long-term ERT use conferred more protection than short-term use, was found in two studies.[22,23] However, ERT users are known to have a different lifestyle than nonusers. ERT users are more health conscious (exercise more, better nutrition) and have higher levels of education than nonusers. These potential confounders may bias the results.[10]

Recently, the results of a study ancillary to the Heart and Estrogen/Progestin Replacement Study were reported.[24] Knee pain and related disability were assessed in a subset of these women at baseline. At the end of this 4-year randomized clinical trial, no differences in pain or disability were found between the women who received placebo or those who were given an estrogen/progestin preparation. However, due to a variety of limitations (all participants had coronary disease; nonspecific knee pain was studied rather than radiographic knee OA), the results of this trial cannot be considered definitive. Estrogen is known to increase BMD in postmenopausal women, and as noted above, high BMD appears to increase the risk of knee OA. However, the interactions among estrogen, BMD, and knee OA are likely to be complex and more research is needed in this area.

Smoking
Two major longitudinal studies of the effect of smoking on the development of knee OA have provided conflicting results.[14,25] Cigarette smoking decreased the risk of radiographic knee OA in the Framingham cohort, and the protective effect was related to the number of cigarettes smoked per day.[14] However in the Chingford Study of middle-aged men and women, no relationship was found between smoking and disease incidence.[25]

Local Risk Factors

Obesity

Obesity is a strong risk factor for knee OA.[10,12] The relationship is stronger for bilateral than unilateral disease and is greater in women than in men. For instance, among women aged 45 to 64 years, the age-adjusted odds ratio (95% CI) for radiographic knee OA was calculated by tertiles of body mass index (BMI). When the highest tertile was compared with the lowest tertile of BMI, the odds ratio for any OA was 6.2 (3.3 to 11.7), for bilateral OA, 18.0 (6.3 to 51.7), and for symptomatic OA, 8.6 (3.3 to 22.5).[12]

Data from the Framingham study have shown that weight change can affect the risk of developing OA (Table 4).[14] Subjects who gained 5 lb or more between the baseline and follow-up clinic visits had an almost fourfold greater risk for incident OA than those who gained or lost less than 5 lb between visits, whereas those who lost more than 5 lb approximately halved their risk.

There is little evidence that the effect of obesity on the development of knee OA is systemic; current evidence suggests that it acts via biomechanical influences. Any increase in body weight increases the load across the weight-bearing knee joint by a force three to seven times greater than the actual weight gain. In addition, knee alignment may affect the impact of body weight on the knee joint. For instance, knees with varus alignment are especially stressed by excess body weight, resulting in more severe medial tibiofemoral OA.[11]

Physical Activity

There is no evidence that participation in light or moderate levels of physical activity throughout the life cycle will increase an individual's risk of developing knee OA.[10,12,27] In a 5-year longitudinal study of 50- to 70-year-old members of the 50-Plus Runners Association in California, runners were neither more likely to show increased incidence of OA nor more rapid progression of existent OA than were a control group matched for age, sex, occupation, and years of education.[28] Similarly, a variety of other studies that considered hours of habitual physical activity or lifetime leisure activity (walking, dancing, cycling, gardening, outdoor sports) found no association with knee OA. However, in the Framingham study, heavy physical activity was strongly associated with incident knee OA (odds ratio, 7.2; 95% CI, 2.5, 20) in a cohort of men and women with a mean age of 70.1 years.[29]

Participation in high-intensity contact sports is strongly linked to development of knee OA in elite athletes. For instance, female runners and tennis players were three times more likely to have tibiofemoral and patellofemoral OA than were age-matched control subjects.[30] Moreover, almost half of a cohort of retired professional soccer players had OA at a mean age of 40.4 years.[31]

Occupational Activity

Men in occupations that require repetitive overuse of the knee joint, for example, carpenters, carpet layers, painters, miners, dock workers, have an increased risk of developing knee OA. Crouching, kneeling, squatting, climbing stairs, and lifting heavy loads all cause abnormal joint loading across the knee joint and can lead to tissue damage. Very few research studies have included women, but all the evidence to date suggests that the risk factors are similar in both men and women.[32]

Research into occupational joint stress is hampered by the difficulty of assessing the actual physical demands required in various occupations and of determining the actual frequency and amount of joint loading. Most of the research is retrospective, and, thus, the results could be biased.

Injury

Kellgren and Lawrence[33] first described an association between joint injury and knee OA in 1958. Several cross-sectional studies and, more recently, longitudinal studies from the United States, United Kingdom, and the Nether-

---

TABLE 4

Relationships of Weight and BMI to Risk of Knee OA Between Framingham Study Visit 18 (1983-1985) and Visit 22 (1992-1993)

	Odds Ratio*
BMI per 5 units	1.6 (1.2, 2.2)
Weight change per 10 lb	1.4 (1.1, 1.8)
Weight change between visits	
Gain = 5 lb	3.8 (0.7, 20.7)
Gain or loss < 5 lb	1.0
Loss = 5 lb	0.5 (0.2, 1.1)

* Odds ratio adjusted for age, sex, smoking, knee injury, physical activity, hand OA, chondrocalcinosis.

Adapted with permission from Felson DT, Zhang Y, Hannan MT, et al: Risk factors for incident radiographic knee osteoarthritis in the elderly: The Framingham Study. *Arthritis Rheum* 1997;40:728-733.

---

lands have confirmed that knee injury (defined as any knee injury that prevented unaided walking for at least a week) is a strong predictor for the development of knee OA.[10,11]

In 1990 it was estimated that the annual incidence of knee ligament injury in the United States was 98 per 100,000, with resultant knee instability in about two thirds of the injured cohort. Most knee injuries involve the anterior cruciate ligament (ACL), and ACL rupture is often associated with meniscal damage or a tear in the medial collateral ligament. Both ACL deficiency and meniscal rupture are strongly linked to early degenerative arthritic changes.[34,35] It is not clear to what extent ACL reconstruction can delay the onset of arthritis but results of one relatively small (n = 53) recent study suggest that early ACL reconstruction with meniscal preservation provides the greatest protection during a 7-year follow-up period. The poorest postoperative outcomes were seen following meniscectomy.[36] Additional research is needed to study the long-term effect of ACL injury, reconstructive techniques, and timing of surgical intervention on the development of arthritic changes.

Mechanical Environment of the Joint

Epidemiologic and clinical research has begun to focus on the way in which specific characteristics of the knee joint (alignment, proprioception, ligamentous laxity) may influence the development of arthritic changes.[10,11] Knee alignment (the position of the knee relative to the hip and ankle) has a strong influence on load distribution across the knee joint. Varus alignment is associated with progressive medial OA (assessed by joint space narrowing) and valgus alignment with lateral OA. The degree of malalignment is correlated with the magnitude of joint space narrowing.[37]

Proprioception, which helps to establish and maintain joint stability, is decreased in both the involved and uninvolved knees of patients with unilateral knee OA when compared with proprioception in age-matched control subjects. These data suggest that loss of proprioceptive accuracy may occur before pathology develops, but the mechanisms are not clear.[11]

Knee laxity, or instability, also affects joint mechanics. Varus-valgus laxity increases with age and on average is greater in women than men. It has been shown that patients with unilateral knee OA have greater varus-valgus laxity in both the involved and contralateral knees than age-matched control subjects. Thus it appears that

increased laxity may precede the development of knee OA.[11,38]

Muscle Strength

Loss of muscle strength in the lower extremities is strongly associated with joint disorders and disability, and it is well established that many patients with knee OA have quadriceps weakness.[10,11,39] Originally it was assumed that this decreased muscle strength was the result of disuse atrophy secondary to knee pain. But newer studies[39,40] have shown that this extensor weakness is present in women with asymptomatic tibiofemoral OA, suggesting that quadriceps weakness is a risk factor for knee OA. In a study of subjects with no evidence of knee OA at the time of enrollment, the women with knee OA during the follow-up period had 18% lower quadriceps strength at baseline than the women who remained free of OA. No such relationship was found in men. However, in this study muscle strength did not influence disease progression in either men or women.[11]

RISK FACTORS FOR PROGRESSION OF KNEE OSTEOARTHRITIS

Measurement of joint space narrowing (JSN) is currently the recommended method for monitoring disease progression in knee OA. This method has been shown to be more sensitive to change than use of the Kellgren and Lawrence grading system. Joint space narrowing is measured directly and also assessed using the Altman atlas and categorized on a four-point scale (0 = none, 1 = possible, 2 = definite, and 3 = severe).[41]

Patients with knee OA rarely show evidence of radiographic improvement, and many remain stable over long periods. Between 3% and 12% of patients progress each year, and the mean annual decrease in joint space ranges from 0.18 to 0.60 mm. The rate of disease progression is highly variable.

More research is needed to better define the risk factors for disease progression. Current evidence suggests that obesity and contralateral knee OA are the strongest predictive factors. Low dietary intake of vitamins C and D may also play an important role. A recent study by Sharma and associates[37] reported that tibiofemoral OA progresses asymmetrically. Subjects with varus alignment were found to have a threefold greater risk (adjusted for age, sex, and BMI) for progression in the medial compartment than

Adapted with permission from Wolfe F, Lane NE. The longterm outcome of osteoarthritis: Rates and predictors of joint space narrowing in symptomatic patients with knee osteoarthritis. *J Rheumatol* 2002;29:139-146.

TABLE 5

Rate of Progression to Maximum JSN Score According to First Knee Radiograph for Patients with Knee OA

JSN at First Observation	Number of Patients	Incidence Rate (%)	50% Survival Time (years)
0	583	1.7	17.84
1	434	3.2	12.03
2	215	7.7	7.44

did subjects with neutral or mild valgus (≤ 2°) alignment. Similarly, valgus alignment conferred a threefold greater risk for lateral compartment progression during an 18-month follow-up period.

RISK FACTORS FOR PAIN

Relatively little is known about the etiology of pain associated with knee OA.[3,10] Most individuals with radiographic evidence of knee OA do not report pain on most days during the month. However, as radiographic severity increases so also does the risk of reporting pain. In addition, a variety of psychological factors (depression, anxiety, coping style) may be associated with painful symptoms in patients with knee OA.[42]

RISK FACTORS FOR DISABILITY

Disability attributed to knee OA is greater than that caused by any other medical condition in the elderly but it is not known how the disease process causes disability.[3,43] To date, research has shown only a weak relationship between disease severity (assessed radiographically) and disability. This result may reflect limitations in evaluating both disease severity and disability in the studies. Use of more sophisticated techniques, such as MRI, in epidemiologic studies may provide new insights into the pathoanatomic and pathophysiologic factors associated with disability.[10,43]

Pain is a major determinant of loss of physical function in persons with knee OA. Difficulty with ambulation and

transfer occur two to three times more frequently among men and women with symptomatic OA than among those with asymptomatic disease. However, several studies have also shown that severe radiographic asymptomatic OA is more likely to be associated with reduced lower extremity functioning than is less severe symptomatic OA.[2,44-46] Thus the relationships between pain, disability, and disease severity appear to be complex.

Functional impairment in patients with knee OA is also associated with reduced quadriceps strength and a variety of psychological factors, such as depression, anxiety, pain coping, and self-efficacy.

RISK FACTORS FOR PROGRESSION TO KNEE ARTHROPLASTY

When medical treatment fails to alleviate the symptoms of severe OA, arthroplasty may be considered. Although symptoms of pain and disability are not closely associated with radiographic changes, patients do not become candidates for knee arthroplasty unless severe JSN is evident, that is, JSN = 3.

In a recently published long-term study of patients with knee pain, Wolfe and Lane[47] determined the time it took to reach a JSN score of three. It took 17.84 years for 50% of patients with normal joint space on entry into the study (JSN = 0) to progress to JSN = 3; 12.03 years for 50% of those entering with JSN = 1; and 7.44 years for 50% of those entering with JSN = 2 (Table 5). The strongest risk factor for progression to maximum narrowing was severity of JSN at first observation. Obesity and symptom duration before enrollment in the study were weaker predictors. The presence of radiographic abnormalities in the contralateral knee was predictive of progression only among the patients with JSN = 0 at the beginning of the study.

Both hip and knee arthroplasty are cost-effective and improve the quality of life for patients. However, because arthroplasty is an elective procedure, patient preferences affect the decision to proceed. It has been shown that only 8% to 15% of patients with a demonstrated need (based on symptoms and radiographic evidence) are willing to undergo the procedure. Younger patients (aged 55 to 64 years) were twice as likely to seriously consider arthroplasty than were other patients. Discussion with their physicians was also a positive predictor. Neither symptom severity nor sex predicted willingness to have surgery.[48]

Summary

Knee OA, once considered an inevitable consequence of aging, is now recognized to be multifactorial, resulting from the interaction of a variety of systemic and local factors, including age, genetic predisposition, obesity, trauma, and mechanical properties of the synovial joint. However, in spite of intensive research during the past 20 years, very little is known about the onset and progression of the disease. A new US national research program, the Osteoarthritis Initiative, will focus on identifying biomarkers that signal the onset or progression of knee OA. These biomarkers may help to identify persons with early subclinical changes in bony or soft tissue and those at risk for progressive disease. Such quantitative monitoring of the disease process will allow clinicians to better assess the effectiveness of drug therapy and manage their patients on an individualized basis.

Bibliography

1. Dunlop DD, Manheim LM, Yelin EH, Song J, Chang RW: The costs of arthritis. *Arthritis Rheum* 2003;49:101-113.

2. Keuttner KE, Goldberg VM: Introduction, in Keuttner KE, Goldberg VM (eds): *Osteoarthritic Disorders*. Rosemont, IL, American Academy of Orthopaedic Surgeons, 1995, pp xxi-xxv.

3. Klippel JH, Crofford LJ, Stone JH, Weyand CM (eds): *Primer on the Rheumatic Diseases*, ed 12. Atlanta, GA, Arthritis Foundation, 2001.

4. Kellgren JH, Lawrence JS: Radiological assessment of osteoarthrosis. *Arthritis Rheum Dis* 1957;16:494-501.

5. Anderson JJ, Felson DT: Factors associated with osteoarthritis of the knee in the first national Health and Nutrition Examination Survey (HANES I): Evidence for an association with overweight, race, and physical demands of work. *Am J Epidemiol* 1988;128:179-189.

6. Jordan JM, Linder GF, Renner JB, Fryer JG: The impact of arthritis in rural populations. *Arthr Care Res* 1995;8:242-250.

7. Yoshida S, Aoyagi K, Felson DT, Aliabadi P, Shind H, Takemoto T: Comparison of the prevalence of radiographic osteoarthritis of the knee and hand between Japan and the United States. *J Rheumatol* 2002;29:1454-1458.

8. Zhang Y, Xu L, Nevitt MC, et al: Comparison of the prevalence of knee osteoarthritis between the elderly Chinese population in Beijing and whites in the United States: The Beijing Osteoarthritis Study. *Arthritis Rheum* 2001;44:2065-2071.

9. Oliveria SA, Felson D, Reed J, et al: Incidence of symptomatic hand, hip, and knee osteoarthritis among patients in a health maintenance organization. *Arthritis Rheum* 1995;38:1134-1141.

10. Felson DT: Lawrence RA, Dieppe PA, et al: Osteoarthritis: New insights. Part 1: The disease and its risk factors. *Ann Intern Med* 2000;133:635-646.

11. Sharma L: Local factors in osteoarthritis. *Curr Opin Rheumatol* 2001;13:441-446.

12. Sowers MF: Epidemiology of risk factors for osteoarthritis: Systemic factors. *Curr Opin Rheumatol* 2001;13:447-451.

13. Simonet WS: Genetics of primary generalized osteoarthritis. *Mol Genet Metab* 2002;77:31-34.

14. Felson DT, Zhang Y, Hannan MT, et al: Risk factors for incident radiographic knee osteoarthritis in the elderly: The Framingham Study. *Arthritis Rheum* 1997;40:728-733.

15. Lane NE, Nevitt MC: Osteoarthritis, bone mass and fractures: How are they related? *Arthritis Rheum* 2002;46:1-4.

16. Zhang Y, Hannan MT, Chaisson CE, et al: Bone mineral density and risk of incident and progressive radiographic knee osteoarthritis in women: The Framingham Study. *J Rheumatol* 2000;27:1032-1037.

17. Hart DJ, Cronin C, Daniels M, Worthy T, Doyle DV, Spector TD: The relationship of bone density and fracture to incident and progressive radiographic osteoarthritis of the knee: The Chingford Study. *Arthritis Rheum* 2002;46:92-99.

18. Nevitt MC, Felson DT: Sex hormones and the risk of osteoarthritis in women: Epidemiological evidence. *Ann Rheum Dis* 1996;9:673-676.

19. Felson DT, Nevitt MC: Estrogen and osteoarthritis: How do we explain conflicting study results? *Preventive Med* 1999;28:445-448.

20. Spector TD, Nandra D, Hart DJ, Doyle DV: Is hormone replacement protective for hand and knee osteoarthritis in women? The Chingford Study. *Ann Rheum Dis* 1997;56:432-434.

21. Sandmark H, Hogstedt C, Lewold S, Vingard E: Osteoarthrosis of the knee in men and women in association with overweight, smoking, and hormone therapy. *Ann Rheum Dis* 1999;58151-155.

22. Hannan MT, Felson DT, Anderson JJ, Naimark A, Kannel WB: Estrogen use and radiographic arthritis of the knee in women: The Framingham Osteoarthritis Study. *Arthritis Rheum* 1990;33:525-532.

23. Nevitt MC, Cummings ST, Lane NE, et al: Association of estrogen replacement therapy with the risk of osteoarthritis in elderly women. *Arch Intern Med* 1996;156:2073-2080.

24. Nevitt MD, Felson DT, Williams EN, Grady D: The effect of estrogen plus progestin on knee symptoms and related disability in postmenopausal women: The Heart and Estrogen/Progestin Replacement Study. A randomized

double-blind placebo-controlled trial. *Arthritis Rheum* 2001;44:811-818.

25. Hart DJ, Doyle DV, Spector TD: Association between metabolic factors and knee osteoarthritis in middle-aged women: The Chingford Study. *Arthritis Rheum* 1999;42:17-24.

26. Hart DJ, Spector TD: The relationship of obesity, fat distribution and osteoarthritis in women in the general population: The Chingford Study. *J Rheumatol* 1993;20:331-335.

27. Buckwalter JA, Lane NE: Athletics and osteoarthritis. *Am J Sports Med* 1997;25:873-881.

28. Lane NE, Michel B, Bjorken A, et al: The risk of osteoarthritis with running and aging: A 5-year longitudinal study. *J Rheumatol* 1993;20:461-468.

29. McAlindon TE, Wilson PW, Aliabadi P, et al: Level of physical activity and risk of radiographic and symptomatic knee osteoarthritis in the elderly: The Framingham Study. *Am J Med* 1999;106:151-157.

30. Spector TD, Harris PA, Hart DJ, et al: Risk of osteoarthritis associated with long-term weight-bearing sports. *Arthritis Rheum* 1996;39:988-995.

31. Turner AP, Barlow JH, Heathcote-Elliott C: Long term impact of playing professional football in the United Kingdom. *Brit J Sports Med* 2000;34:332-336.

32. Schauten JS, de Bie RA, Swaen G: An update on the relationship between occupational factors and osteoarthritis of the hip and knee. *Curr Opin Rheumatol* 2002;14:89-92.

33. Kellgren JH, Lawrence JS: Osteoarthritis and disc degeneration in an urban population. *Ann Rheum Dis* 1958;17:388-396.

34. Gelber AC, Hochberg MC, Mead LA, Wang NY, Wigley FM, Klag MJ: Joint injury in young adults and risk for subsequent hip and knee osteoarthritis. *Ann Intern Med* 2000;133:321-328.

35. Gillquist J, Messner K: Anterior cruciate ligament reconstruction and long term incidence of gonarthrosis. *Sports Med* 1999;27:143-156.

36. Jomha NM, Borton DC, Clingeleffer AJ, Pinczewski LA: Long-term arthritic changes in anterior cruciate ligament reconstructed knees. *Clin Orthop* 1999;358:188-193.

37. Sharma L, Song J, Felson DT, Cahue S, Shamiyeh E, Dunlop DD: The role of knee alignment in disease progression and functional decline in knee osteoarthritis. *JAMA* 2001;286:188-195.

38. Sharma L, Lou C, Felson DT, et al: Laxity in healthy and osteoarthritic knees. *Arthritis Rheum* 1999;42:861-870.

39. Slemenda C, Heilman DK, Brandt KD, et al: Reduced quadriceps strength relative to body weight: A risk factor for knee osteoarthritis in women? *Arthritis Rheum* 1998;41:1951-1959.

40. Hurley MV: The role of muscle weakness in the pathogenesis of osteoarthritis. *Rheum Dis Clin North Am* 1999;25:283-298.

41. Altman RD, Hochberg MC, Murphey WA Jr, Wolfe F, Lequesne M: Atlas of individual radiographic features in osteoarthritis. *Osteoarthritis Cartilage* 1995;3:3070

42. van Baar ME, Dekker J, Lemmens JA, Oostendorp RA, Bijlsma JW: Pain and disability in patients with osteoarthritis of hip or knee: The relationship with articular, kinesiological, and psychological characteristics. *J Rheumatol* 1998;25:125-133.

43. Sharma L, Lou C, Felson DT, et al: Laxity in healthy and osteoarthritic knees. *Arthritis Rheum* 1999;42:861-870.

44. Rejeski WJ, Craven T, Ettinger WH, McFarlane M, Shumaker S: Self efficacy and pain in disability with osteoarthritis of the knee. *J Gerontol B Psychol Sci Soc Sci 1* 1995;51:P24-P29.

45. Ling SM, Fried LP, Garett Es, Fan MY, Rantanen T, Bathon JM: Knee osteoarthritis compromises early mobility function: The Women's Health and Aging Study II. *J Rheumatol* 2003;30:114-120.

46. Bruyere O, Honore A, Rovati LC, et al: Radiologic features poorly predict clinical outcomes in knee osteoarthritis. *Scand J Rheumatol* 2002;31:13-16.

47. Wolfe F, Lane NE: The longterm outcome of osteoarthritis: Rates and predictors of joint space narrowing in symptomatic patients with knee osteoarthritis. *J Rheumatol* 2002;29:139-146.

48. Hawker GA, Wright JG, Coyte PC, et al: Determining the need for hip and knee arthroplasty: The role of clinical severity and patients' preferences. *Med Care* 2001;39:206-216.

CHAPTER 2

FLUID REPLACEMENT AND ARTHROSCOPIC DÉBRIDEMENT IN THE TREATMENT OF OSTEOARTHRITIS

MOISÉS COHEN, MD
RENE JORGE ABDALLA, MD
BENNO EJNISMAN, MD
JOICEMAR AMARO, MD

Osteoarthritis (OA) is the most prevalent form of arthritis in the world. Approximately 6% of the population of the United States older than 30 years is affected; of these, 65% have frequent knee pain that is attributed to OA.[1] Clinically, patients with OA report pain that is worse with weight bearing and improved with rest, decreased range of motion, and diminished quality of life. Physical examination often reveals tenderness, crepitus, bony enlargement, and limited joint motion.

Chondral lesions can be treated in many ways, with physiotherapy, pharmacologic therapy, or surgery; however, no one approach is considered a "gold standard," because the properties of cartilage are almost impossible to reproduce. The goals of treatment are symptom relief, maintenance of an active lifestyle, and delayed surgical treatment. If surgical treatment is considered, several factors must be examined, including minimal morbidity risk, cost, type of procedure, and potential for early rehabilitation, measurable outcomes, and good long-term results.

Nonsurgical treatment should be tried first, particularly in active, middle-age patients. Orthopaedists should be skilled in early diagnosis of OA and familiar with current, common nonsurgical treatments, including patient education, hydrotherapy, strengthening and stretching programs, activity and shoe modifications, and brace treatments. Patients who are overweight should be encouraged to participate in a comprehensive weight management program, including dietary counseling and aerobic exercise.

Surgical treatment, specifically total knee arthroplasty (TKA), has been shown to have good results at both short- and long-term follow-up; however, postoperatively, patients' anatomy is permanently altered, and patients often limit their activities and experience complications, which can result in a poor prognosis. Thus, another point to consider is that because middle-aged patients are more active than in the past, TKA should not be considered first.

Arthroscopic osteochondral autograft transplantation is also often used to treat chondral/osteochondral lesions of the femoral condyle, but this technique is expensive and technically difficult. There are no randomized prospective studies that compare the natural history of the repair tissue to that of other forms of repair tissue, and long-term functional outcomes are still relatively unknown. In addition, autologous chondrocyte implantation has not been shown to prevent degenerative changes. During the past decade, however, several competing techniques have evolved to stimulate articular cartilage repair. When the damaged area is more extensive, osteochondral cylinder grafting (mosaicplasty) should be considered.

FLUID REPLACEMENT

The healthy human knee joint contains about 2 mL of synovial fluid. Hyaluronic acid is present in the synovial fluid at a concentration of 2 to 3 mg/mL. This molecule binds to proteoglycan to form macromolecular aggregates. In the arthritic knee, synovial fluid is more abundant and viscous; the hyaluronic acid concentration is decreased by one third to one half, and the molecular size is reduced. These alterations severely decrease (1) shock absorption, (2) dissipation and storage of energy caused by trauma, and (3) lubrication of the protective coating of the articular cartilage surface.

Viscosupplementation

To restore the concentration of synovial fluid, the concept of viscosupplementation was introduced as a solution to the problems associated with OA of the knee.[2] Its efficacy in the knee (just as in the hip and shoulder), however, appears to decrease over time.

Injection

Intra-articular injections are often tried to limit the use of nonsteroidal anti-inflammatory drugs and to delay surgery, but results vary depending on the product used. Roman and associates[3] concluded that the best course of action appears to be one injection a week for 5 weeks, during which time the joint eliminates the excess hyaluronic acid. In their study, treatment was reported to be well tolerated with no serious adverse reactions or changes in blood or urine values. Adverse effects consisted of transient pain, occasionally accompanied by warmth, that usually lasted no longer than 1 to 2 days before spontaneous resolution. The authors also reported good to excellent immediate results in 41% of their patients, but after 6 months, almost three quarters of their patients reported only a fair result or no clinical response.

Miltner and associates[4] conducted a prospective controlled study of 43 patients with OA to evaluate the effectiveness of injection at reducing symptoms. The treatment group received an intra-articular injection in the affected knee once a week for 5 weeks, while the control group was injected in the opposite, unaffected knee in the same manner. The treatment group reported pain relief and functional improvement, evidenced by increased total work of the knee flexors and extensors on isokinetic machines. Patient reports using the visual analog scale revealed that pain was reduced at rest and during weight-bearing tests. No studies mentioned joint infection as a result of injection.[2]

ARTHROSCOPIC LAVAGE AND DÉBRIDEMENT

The use of the arthroscope dates back to 1934 when Burman and associates reported improved symptoms in 10 patients who were treated with arthroscopic lavage. However, their study was simply a collection of case reports reviewed retrospectively. Since then, the role of arthroscopy in the treatment of OA of the knee has been subject to continuous change, as have the expectations of surgeons and patients. Arthroscopic débridement has

PERSONAL EXPERIENCE

Study design Single-center, randomized, prospective study; the preoperative VAS was > 60 for pain and activities of daily living.

Patient characteristics A total of 116 patients (77 male and 39 female); age 38 to 58 years old (mean, 48.4 years)

Follow-up evaluation 26, 52, and 104 weeks

Outcomes measures Pain and activities daily of living

Results Improvement rate of 63% at 26 weeks, 54% at 52 weeks, and 20% 104 weeks

Conclusion Arthroscopic lavage and débridement provide positive outcomes, but symptom reduction is often short-lived. This approach may be indicated to reduce symptoms before a more major procedure (eg, TKA) is considered.

PERSONAL EXPERIENCE

Study design Single-center, randomized, prospective study; preoperative VAS was > 60 for pain and activities of daily living.

Patient selection A total of 513 patients/532 knees (385 male and 128 female); age 39 to 59 years (mean, 49.6 years)

Follow-up 2 to 16 years (mean, 9.3 years)

Outcomes measures Pain and activities of daily living

Results Three groups (213 abrasion, 251 drilling, 68 microfracture technique)of patients were followed at 2 and 5 years. Improvement was reported in 63% of patients at 2 to 5 years; in 38% of patients at 5 to 10 years, but in only 9% at more than 10 years. The difference between drilling and microfracture technique was not significantly different, whereas results of abrasion procedures were associated to the worst results after 5 years. A "second-look" arthroscopy and biopsy were performed in 28 patients, all associated with some new procedure; of these, 6 were done between 2 and 5 years' follow-up, 14 between 5 and 10 years, and 8 after more than 10 years. There was no detectable hyaline cartilage tissue in any of these patients, even in those with longer follow-up; in all cases, the biopsy specimen showed fibrocartilage tissue.

Conclusion All three procedures resulted in temporary benefit and can be considered reasonable alternatives before TKA in active, middle-age patients.

become a commonly performed procedure, but careful patient selection is mandatory. The results of many arthroscopic procedures are quite encouraging with early follow-up, with an ultimate goal to prevent long-term degenerative arthritis.[5,7,8]

Patient selection should depend of many factors; according to Harwin,[9] younger patients do somewhat better than older patients, and patients with larger angular deformities do worse than those with less deviation. Patients who had prior meniscectomy were also shown to do less well. The ideal patient had less than 5° of angular deformity. The author reported good results in 63% of patients (mean follow-up, 7.4 years).

Lavage removes microscopic and macroscopic fragments of cartilage and loose bodies that may result in synovitis, which is a likely source of knee pain. Lavage also removes calcium phosphate crystals that are detectable in most severe cases of OA in the knee. This technique probably works because degradative enzymes, which contribute to synovitis and to the further breakdown of articular cartilage, are removed.[6] Livesley and associates[14] compared the efficacy of lavage and physiotherapy with that of physiotherapy alone. At the 1-year follow-up, the group that received lavage with physiotherapy reported better pain relief than the other group.

Débridement consists of smoothing rough, fibrillated articular and meniscal surfaces and shaving tibial spine osteophytes that interfere with range of motion. The surgeon should be conservative when using this technique, however, removing only fibrillated and scaling fragments of articular cartilage.[7]

Fond and associates[10] evaluated 2- and 5-year results of 36 patients who underwent arthroscopic débridement. Approximately 70% of patients had tibial osteophytes anteromedial to the anterior tibial spine, which contributed to their diminished knee extension. At the 2-year follow-up, 89% of their patients reported good to excellent results. However, the results deteriorated over time. At the 5-year mark, only 69% of patients reported good or excellent results. The presence of tricompartmental disease was predictive of poor results. Patients with preop-

FIGURE 1

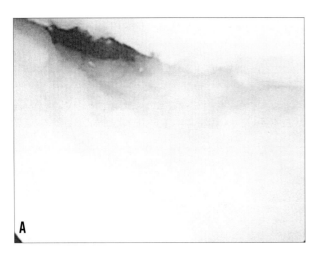 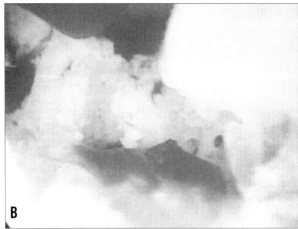

Arthroscopic view of a chondral lesion of the femoral trochlea. **A**, After abrasion. **B**, After release of the tourniquet, bleeding from the subchondral bone is seen.

erative flexion contractures of less than 10° and preoperative Hospital for Special Surgery scores greater than 22 benefited from arthroscopic débridement.

Patient age should be considered as an important factor when considering arthroscopic débridement. Way and associates[11] reviewed 14,391 eligible patients who underwent unilateral arthroscopic knee débridement. Overall, 9.2% of patients required TKA 1 year after débridement, and 18.4% required TKA within 3 years. Patients who were at least 70 years old were 4.7 times more likely to undergo an early TKA.

The presence of severe (grade IV) chondromalacia was associated with subsequent surgery and when the medial compartment or bicondylar disease was involved, the likelihood of a poor outcome increased significantly.[12] McGinley and associates[13] showed that knees (37%) with Outerbridge grade IV changes in 80% of one compartment did not require TKA after 10 years' follow-up. The authors, however, selected only those patients who had undergone arthroscopy as a temporizing procedure. Of these patients, 67% did not undergo TKA at an average of 13.2 years follow-up.

Moseley and associates[15] conducted a randomized, placebo-controlled trial to evaluate the efficacy of arthroscopy for OA. A total of 180 patients received arthroscopic débridement, lavage, or placebo surgery. Patients in the placebo surgery group received skin incisions and underwent a simulated débridement without insertion of the arthroscope. At no point did either of the intervention groups report less pain or better function than the placebo surgery group. Although recent prospective, randomized, double-blind studies have demonstrated that outcomes after arthroscopic lavage or débridement were no better than a placebo procedure for knee OA, controversy still exists. With proper selection, patients with early OA and mechanical symptoms of locking or catching can benefit from arthroscopic surgery.[16]

Postoperative rehabilitation should be tailored to the patient, given the findings at surgery, rather than adhere to a rigid protocol. In general, early range of motion should be encouraged to prevent venous thrombosis. In particular, synovectomies and chondroplasties performed in the weight-bearing area of the joint or in the patellofemoral compartment can be extremely uncomfortable, and a cane or crutches may be necessary for a few days after surgery.[7] The use of hydrotherapy and kinesitherapy are very important postoperatively, and patients should gradually return to full activities 1 to 2 months postoperatively.

ABRASION, DRILLING, AND MICROFRACTURE TECHNIQUE

The biologic resurfacing of a joint under arthroscopic control is the challenge facing orthopaedic surgeons today.

Healing and restoration of articular tissues to some functional biologic state seems to be a reasonable goal (Figure 1).

Results of arthroscopic chondroplasty are unpredictable. Concerns include the durability of the fibrocartilage repair tissue in subchondral penetration procedures and thermal damage to subchondral bone and adjacent normal articular cartilage in laser/thermal chondroplasty.

Débridement, drilling, microfracture technique, and abrasion chondroplasty have been shown to result in fibrocartilage with inferior mechanical properties when compared with hyaline cartilage (Figure 2). No long-term studies have been published to confirm the benefits of replacing osteochondral defects with hyaline cartilage rather than fibrocartilage.

REFERENCES

1. Felson D, Buckwalter J: Debridement and lavage for osteoarthritis of the knee. *N Engl J Med* 2002;347:132-133.

2. Peyron JG: Intraarticular hyaluronan injections in the treatment of osteoarthritis: State-of-art review. *J Reumatol* 1993;20:10-15.

3. Roman JA, Chismol J, Morales M, Donderis JL: Intra-articular treatment with hyaluronic acid. Comparative study of hyalgan and adant. *Clin Reumatol* 2000;19:204-206.

4. Miltner O, Schneider U, Siebert CH, Niedhart C, Niedthard FU: Efficacy of intraarticular hyaluronic acid in patients with osteoarthritis: A prospective clinical trial. *Osteoarthritis Cartilage* 2002;10:680-686.

5. Cain EL, Clancy WG: Treatment algorithm for osteochondral injuries of the knee. *Clin Sports Med* 2001;20:321-342.

6. Gilbert JE: Current treatment options for the restoration of articular cartilage. *Am J Knee Surg* 1998;11:42-46.

7. Fu FH, Harner CD, Vince KG: *Knee Surgery.* pp 1113-1120.

8. Jackson RW, Dieterichs C: The results of arthroscopic lavage and débridement of osteoarthritic knees based on the based of degeneration: A 4 to 6 years symptomatic follow-up. *Arthroscopy* 2003;19:13-20.

9. Harwin SF: Arthroscopic débridement for osteoarthritis of the knee: Predictors of patient satisfaction. *Arthroscopy* 1999;15:142-146.

10. Fond J, Rodin D, Ahmad S, Nirschl RP: Arthroscopic débridement for the treatment of osteoarthritis in the knee 2-and 5-years follow-up. *Arthroscopy* 2002;18:829-834.

FIGURE 2

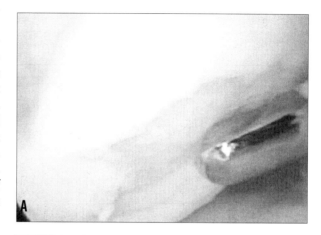

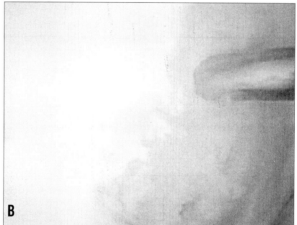

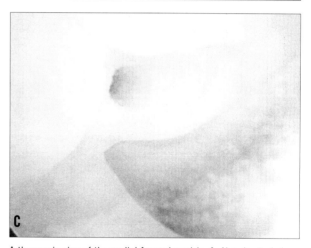

Arthroscopic view of the medial femoral condyle. **A**, Abrasion technique using a shaver. **B**, Drilling technique using a Kirschner wire. **C**, Microfracture technique.

11. Way EK, Kreder HJ, Williams J: Arthroscopic débridement of the knee for osteoarthritis in patients fifty years of age or older: Utilization and outcomes the province of Ontario. *J Bone Joint Surg Am* 2002;84:17-22.

12. Ogilvie-Harris DJ, Fitsalos DP: Arthroscopic management of the degenerative knee. *Arthroscopy* 1991;17:151-157.

13. McGinley BJ, Cushner FD, Scott WN: Débridement arthroscopy 10 years follow-up. *Clin Orthop* 1999;367:190-194.

14. Livesley PJ, Doherty M, Needoff M, Moulton A: Arthroscopic lavage of osteoarthritic knees. *J Bone Joint Surg Br* 1991;73:922-926.

15. Moseley JB, O'Malley K, Petersen NJ, Terri J, Brody BA, Kuykendall DH, Hollingsworth JC, Ashton CM, Wray NP: A controlled trial of arthroscopic surgery for osteoarthritis of the knee. *N Engl J Med* 2002;347:81-88.

16. Hunt SA, Jazrawi LM, Sherman OH: Arthroscopic management of osteoarthritis of the knee. *J Am Acad Orthop Surg* 2002;10:356-363.

CHAPTER 3

OSTEOTOMIES ABOUT THE KNEE

GIANCARLO PUDDU, MD
VITTORIO FRANCO, MD
MASSIMO CIPOLLA, MD
GUGLIELMO CERULLO, MD
ENRICO GIANNI, MD

Medial compartment osteoarthritis (OA) and varus deformity are very common knee conditions in the general population. Degenerative genu valgum is a less frequent but very disabling condition. Thus, varus and valgus deformities of the lower extremity play an important role in OA of the knee. Malalignment into a varus position overloads the medial condyles of the femur and tibia, whereas valgus malalignment overloads the lateral condyles. Degenerative changes of the articular cartilage are highly related to the forces exerted on the bearing surfaces and can occur through tension, compression, or shear. Specific trauma and trauma from the overload caused by obesity or occupational factors are etiologically important, and genetic factors are also known to play a part. However, the biophysical cause of OA is an overload or a concentration of forces, strictly related to the limb alignment, beyond the coping ability of the cartilage and subchondral bone.

In any discussion of OA of the knee and its treatment,

One or more of the authors or the departments with which they are affiliated have received something of value from a commercial or other party related directly or indirectly to the subject of this chapter.

the subject of arthroplasty versus osteotomy is always pertinent. Historically, osteotomy preceded arthroplasty by about 10 years. As arthroplasty became more common in the 1970s, the indication for each operation clarified. The number of osteotomies performed each year has remained almost stable, but the proportional rate of total knee arthroplasties (TKA) has increased dramatically in recent years.

The rationale behind the osteotomy is to correct the angular deformity at the knee, thereby decreasing the excessive weight-bearing load across the affected compartment where the degenerative process is greatest. Since alternative treatments for severe OA of the knee were limited in the 1960s, tibial osteotomy was used initially for OA, rheumatoid arthritis, and secondary arthritis, regardless of the etiopathogenesis and the magnitude of the angular deformity. After several years' experience, Coventry,[1] Insall and associates,[2] and others narrowed the indications for tibial osteotomy. By the late 1970s, high tibial osteotomy was being used for younger, more active patients in whom TKA was thought to be ill-advised.

Today, patients selected for proximal tibial/distal femoral osteotomy typically have unicompartmental OA with axial malalignment. However, fracture, trauma, congenital and acquired deformities, and idiopathic osteonecrosis are also indications for osteotomy.

INDICATIONS AND CONTRAINDICATIONS

There is no definite chronologic age below which an osteotomy is indicated and above which an arthroplasty is indicated. The age 65 is most often cited, but activity level, lifestyle, and general health must be considered. As long-term studies of arthroplasty will demonstrate, age considerations may change. But the fact still remains that osteotomy patients are generally younger than candidates for arthroplasty.

Osteotomy is best reserved for patients with unicompartmental OA with generally well-maintained knee range of motion of at least 90° of flexion and less than 15° of flexion contracture. Osteotomy probably should not be performed in patients with rheumatoid arthritis or very unstable knees because, according to Insall and associates,[3] these patients likely have severe ligamentous laxity and subluxation. In knees with greater than 20° of varus deformity or 15° of valgus deformity, osteotomy is contraindicated.

A medial or lateral meniscectomy that leads to a symptomatic deformity is also a frequent indication for an osteotomy. Too often, the meniscus is sacrificed in young athletes who undergo a surgical procedure after a sprain of the knee. In these patients, timing of reparative surgery is very important because an osteotomy is much more effective if performed in the earliest stage of the condition. This prevents late, unavoidable degenerative changes in the joint of still young, active patients. Similarly, a young patient with a painful congenital deformity can be considered a candidate for an early preventive osteotomy before articular damage starts to involve the overloaded compartment.

A patient with a varus deformity and anterior cruciate ligament (ACL) insufficiency eventually may be treated with proximal tibial osteotomy in addition to the ACL reconstruction. A technically demanding procedure, the osteotomy associated with the ligament reconstruction addresses the underlying disorder and corrects the problems. Because it is not a routine procedure, it will not be discussed here. However, the symptoms of pain and instability must be separated as clearly as possible because when pain persists, especially in sedentary patients, correction of alignment, with subsequent relief of medial compartment pain, can be a satisfactory treatment.

Obesity is a controversial topic, resulting in conflicting opinions. Obesity has a negative effect on the outcome of surgery in many orthopaedic procedures. While most surgeons would agree that excess body weight may make a patient a better candidate for osteotomy than for arthroplasty, it is also true that obesity represents a negative factor in view of the possible general postoperative complications. When a patient is overweight, steps should be taken to ensure that a more normal weight is achieved prior to surgery to avoid poor long-term results.

A contraindication to osteotomy is severe bone loss (more than 3 to 5 mm) of the medial or lateral tibia or femur. When medial or lateral compartment bony support is insufficient, congruent weight bearing on both tibial plateaus is not possible following the osteotomy. In this situation, tibiofemoral contact will center on the relatively prominent intercondylar tibial spines.

The presence of severe varus or valgus deformity may be associated with lateral or medial subluxation of the tibia, respectively. Subluxation of greater than 1 cm is an absolute contraindication to osteotomy, and some authors suggest that osteotomy should not be performed if any translation or subluxation is present. Studies on the biomechanics of the dynamic gait accurately address the issue of varus or lateral thrust of the knee during ambulation. The term "adductor moment" is used to describe the amount of lateral or varus thrust of the knee observed during gait. Patients with a high adductor moment have poorer results following osteotomy than patients with a low adductor moment. Furthermore, patients with a high adductor moment are more likely to have a recurrent varus deformity following valgus osteotomy. When osteotomy is chosen for those patients despite the presence of a high adductor moment, overcorrection of the deformity may be helpful.

Osteotomy of the proximal tibia or distal femur is designed to relieve pain caused by medial or lateral tibiofemoral OA. Slight degenerative changes of the patellofemoral joint are not a contraindication to osteotomy. However, following proximal tibial osteotomy with a medial opening wedge, the anterior tibial tubercle is lowered at about one half of the angular correction. Therefore, patella baja is a contraindication to this type of procedure.

In summary, we believe that the best indications for tibial or femoral osteotomy are congenital deformity of the knee in a young patient, symptomatic varus or valgus knee with unicompartmental pain, degenerative changes after meniscectomy, and unicompartmental OA. A special indication for proximal tibial osteotomy, combined with or without a reconstruction procedure, is the varus knee with ligamentous laxity and varus thrust.

PREOPERATIVE PLANNING

The weight-bearing line (WBL) is the line connecting the center of the hip and the center of the ankle, passing through the knee and representing the mechanical axis of the knee in the normal morphotype. The femoral anatomic axis coincides with the axis of the shaft, whereas the tibial anatomic axis is also its mechanical axis. The goal of knee osteotomy is to realign the mechanical axis of the limb, thereby shifting the WBL from the diseased compartment to the more normal compartment.

Full-length radiographs of the lower extremity best assess limb alignment. The WBL is a line drawn from the center of the femoral head through the center of the knee to the center of the ankle mortise. The anatomic axis is a line drawn through the center of the femoral and tibial shafts. In the normal knee, the two lines cross in the center of the joint, creating an angle of 5° (physiologic valgus). The mechanical axis, which almost coincides with the WBL, also passes through the center of the joint, or slightly varus (about 1.2° medially).

Using these parameters as the reference points of normal, the deformity is measured. In the varus knee, the WBL is moved through the neutral alignment (approximately the center of the knee) up to a more lateral point at about two thirds (63%) of the tibial plateau to obtain 5° of mechanical valgus alignment, and, therefore, overcorrecting the anatomic valgus from the "normal" 5° to 9° to 10°. Extensive experience has shown that overcorrection is absolutely essential if a good long-standing result from valgus osteotomy is to be achieved. If the osteotomy only corrects the deformity without any overcorrection, it brings the limb axis back to the position from which it originally deformed and does not properly unload the medial compartment. In the normal knee, approximately 60% of weight-bearing forces are transmitted through the medial compartment and approximately 40% through the lateral compartment; even in a severe valgus deformity (up to 30° valgus), the medial plateau load never falls below 30%.

A young patient with a symptomatic congenital varus may be considered an early candidate for a valgus osteotomy; however, overcorrection should be avoided because restoration of the physiologic alignment of the knee will be sufficient.

To reduce the risk of an overcorrection, we prefer to base our planning on a weight-bearing radiograph of both legs as opposed to a radiograph of one leg. The resulting knee deformity, measured on a single-leg stance examination, is the amount of the osseous-geometric malalignment plus the malalignment that results from the ligamentous laxity. The osteotomy realigns the limb by means of a bony correction. The remaining part of the deformity, depending on the ligaments, may recover spontaneously simply because the new balance between the femur and tibia inverts the convex and concave sides of the joint, thereby canceling the effects of the preexisting laxity on varus or valgus alignment.

In a valgus knee, the mechanical axis is repositioned to the neutral alignment at approximately 0° in the center of the joint, resulting in 5° of anatomic and physiologic valgus. The biomechanics of varus and valgus deformities of the knee differ. In fact, the intrinsic valgus angle between the femur and tibia determines an asymmetric overload of the medial compartment, at about 60% of the whole, in the normal knee. Therefore, overbalancing of the knee toward a varus alignment will result in a functional failure because of the additional overload of the medial compartment and the subsequent dramatic acceleration of the degenerative changes of the more normal contralateral side.

The proposed osteotomy is based on the opening wedge technique. Special plates with a spacer "tooth" are designed for this purpose. The plate is chosen based on the size of the base of the wedge, calculated in millimeters. A bigger spacer corresponds to a greater correction, but the correction also depends on the size of the osteotomized bone. The osteotomy must be planned taking into account both the desired correction angle and the size of the tibia at the level of the bone cut.

The WBL method is a simple, reproducible technique for determining the desired correction angle.[4] First, divide the tibial plateau from 0% to 100% from the medial to the lateral margin. Draw two lines, the first one from the center of the femoral head and the second one from the center of the tibiotalar joint to the same point at 63% of the tibial plateau. The angle formed by these two lines is the angle of correction. Once the desired angle of correction is determined, the opening wedge height is calculated by drawing a schematic right triangle in which the apex angle is the one measured with the method described above. One side, the major cathetus, of the triangle is graduated and corresponds to the width of the tibia at the site of the osteotomy; the minor cathetus is the opening base of the wedge. Based on the drawing, it is possible to meas-

FIGURE 1

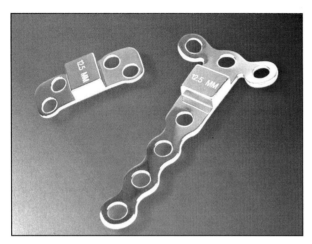

The plates specially designed for this osteotomy are butterfly shaped with four holes for the tibia and "T" shaped with seven holes for the femur.

ure the width of the osteotomy in millimeters to achieve the planned correction with that specific width of the tibia at the site of the osteotomy.

To complete the radiographic evaluation of the knee, lateral and axial views of the patellofemoral joint must be obtained. The Rosenberg view, a posteroanterior weight-bearing radiograph at 45° of knee flexion, facilitates the diagnosis when the AP view is not sensitive enough.[5] The Rosenberg view offers a strong predictive value when the deformity is associated with a cruciate insufficiency and chondral wear is present in the posterior part of the tibial plateaus.

Neither CT nor MRI is recommended for work-up of a candidate for knee osteotomy; however, stress reaction of the subchondral bone, detectable by MRI, could be the only positive sign of a degenerative process at its earlier stage.

DEDICATED SURGICAL INSTRUMENTATION

The object of valgus osteotomy is to obtain a new mechanical axis overcorrected up to 5° of valgus, whereas the purpose of varus osteotomy is to reposition the lower limb to align the physiologic 0° of the neutral mechanical axis. The opening wedge osteotomy is performed with a complete but simple system of dedicated instruments and plates.

Valgus correction of the knee is achieved by means of a proximal tibial osteotomy, and varus correction is achieved by means of distal femoral osteotomy. In a varus deformity, the tibiofemoral joint line is usually parallel to the floor, and the proximal tibial osteotomy has been shown to effectively transfer load from the medial to the lateral compartment. In valgus deformity, the joint line has a valgus tilt with a corresponding obliquity from a supero-lateral to inferomedial direction. While tibial varus osteotomy may realign a valgus limb, it cannot correct the joint line tilt because the procedure is performed distal to the joint. The mechanical consequence in patients with severe valgus deformities (greater than 10° to 12°, according to various authors) is to transfer the load transmission medially not more than the lateral portion of the tibial spine; the resultant increased valgus tilt of the joint line leads to greater shear forces and lateral subluxation during gait. In contrast, a distal femoral varus osteotomy may realign a valgus limb and correct valgus tilt of the joint line when used to treat lateral tibiofemoral OA with valgus deformity.

The specially designed plates for this osteotomy are butterfly shaped with four holes for the tibia and "T" shaped with seven holes for the femur (Figure 1). Their uniqueness is a spacer (tooth) that is available in six different sizes, ranging in thickness from 5 to 17.5 mm (seven sizes up to 20 mm for the femur). Some variations in the shape and dimension of the plate tooth are planned for the future. Tibial plates with trapezoidal spacers also are available to permit correction of the coronal and the so-called tibial posterior slope, and eventually the sagittal deformity, in a single procedure. The new femoral and tibial plates will have the tooth increasing one size for each additional millimeter, from the thinnest to the thickest.

The tooth enters the osteotomic line, holding the position and preventing later bone collapse and recurrence of the deformity. The thickness of the spacer must coincide with the desired angle of correction and must be calculated in advance during the preoperative planning stage. The two upper holes of the tibial plate and the three of the horizontal lower arm of the femoral "T" plate allow the introduction of AO 6.5-mm cancellous screws; the lower holes of the tibial plate and the holes in the vertical arm of the femoral plate are cut for AO 4.5-mm cortical screws.

The crucial point of the procedure is the opening of the metaphysis (where the osteotomy has cut the bone) at the desired angle of correction and holding the position to allow the introduction of the plate tooth. A new and innovative tool, the "osteotomy jack," greatly facilitates this

FIGURE 2

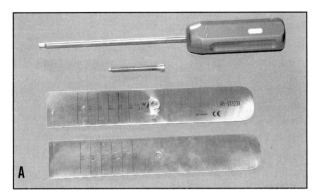

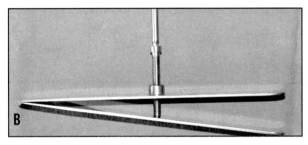

The "osteotomy jack" consists of two osteotomes coupled with a screw long enough to move away the blades and open the osteotomy.

FIGURE 3

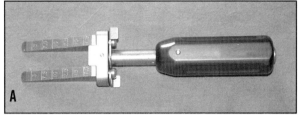

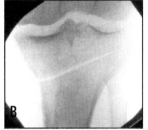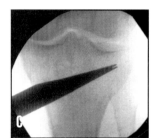

The "wedge opener" enters into the already prepared osteotomy site. It looks like a fork with 2 wedge-shaped tines that are graduated to hold the opening at the correct rate and a removable handle to allow the positioning of the plate.

FIGURE 4

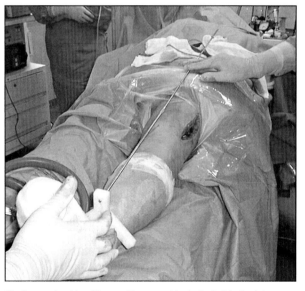

The long rod guide with an ankle support is dedicated to the intraoperative check of the tibiofemoral alignment after the osteotomy.

step. Introduced into the osteotomic line, the jack gently retracts the bone to create a space for the plate and the grafts. It consists of two osteotomes coupled with a screw long enough to move away the blades and open the osteotomy (Figure 2). A very simple "wedge opener" then enters the already prepared osteotomic site. The opener looks like a fork with two wedge-shaped tines, graduated to hold the opening at the correct rate, and a removable handle to allow the positioning of the plate (Figure 3).

The other dedicated tools are the special Homan retractor for the vastus lateralis, to be used in the femoral osteotomy, and a long rod guide with an ankle support to intraoperatively check the mechanical femorotibial alignment (Figure 4).

SURGICAL TECHNIQUE OF TIBIAL OSTEOTOMY

Patient Positioning

On a normal operating table, the patient is in a supine position and the C-arm of an image intensifier is set up opposite to the surgeon. The patient is draped as usual in knee surgery; we also prepare the iliac wing and cover the foot using a very fine stockinette and a transparent adhe-

FIGURE 5

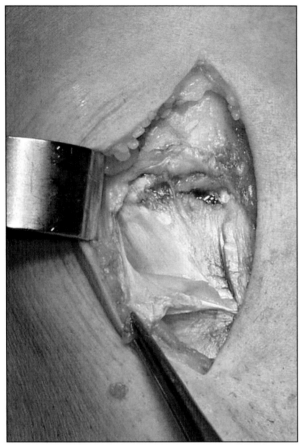

The pes anserinus tendons and the superficial layer of the collateral ligament are carefully dissected and retracted to expose the tibial cortex at the site of the osteotomy.

sive drape to minimize bulging at the ankle so that it will be possible to better realize the femorotibial alignment after the correction. A tourniquet may be inflated.

Arthroscopy

Arthroscopy of the knee is performed before the osteotomy to assess the relative integrity of the contralateral tibiofemoral compartment and patellofemoral joint and to treat any intra-articular pathology; appropriate joint surface débridement, partial meniscectomy, or loose body removal is performed as needed.

Incision and Exposure

The anteromedial aspect of the tibia is exposed through a vertical skin incision centered between the medial border of the anterior tibial tubercle and the anterior edge of the medial collateral ligament, extending 6 to 8 cm distally to the joint line. Sharp dissection is carried to the sartorius fascia, and the pes anserinus tendons are identified and detached from the bone. The pes anserinus is retracted and the anterior half of the underlying superficial collateral ligament is cut horizontally (Figure 5). There is no risk of instability because the deepest and much more stabilizing tibiomeniscal bundle of the ligament remains intact. A blunt retractor is placed dorsally, deep to the collateral ligament, to protect the posterior vessels and expose the posteromedial corner of the tibia. Anteriorly, a second retractor is placed under the patellar tendon. The procedure is facilitated by flexion of the knee.

Osteotomy

Our preferred method is a "free" technique. With the knee in extension and under fluoroscopic control, a Steinmann guide pin is drilled by the "free hand" through the proximal tibia from medial to lateral. This is obliquely oriented, starting approximately 4 cm distal to the joint line and directed across the superior edge of the tibial tubercle to a point 1 cm below the joint line.

The original instruments system also provides an Osteotomy Guide Assembly (ArtroLine AB, Stockholm, Sweden) to assist in the proper placement of the Steinmann guide pin and an Osteotomy Cutting Guide (ArtroLine AB) to facilitate use of the oscillating saw. The guide may be oriented to accommodate variations in size and anatomy; different choices in tilting the osteotomy cut in both coronal and sagittal planes are also possible.

The osteotomy is then performed, keeping the oscillating saw blade below and parallel to the guide pin to prevent an intra-articular fracture. The saw is used to cut the medial cortex only. A sharp osteotome is used to finish the osteotomy, ensuring that all of the cancellous metaphysis and, especially the anterior and the posterior cortices, are completely interrupted but preserving a lateral hinge of approximately 0.5 cm of intact bone (Figure 6). Fibular osteotomy is not necessary.

Wedge Opening

The osteotomic line is easily opened by the help of the jack that gently moves the tibial axis and realigns the knee (Figure 7). The wedge opener is then introduced and slowly advanced into the metaphysis. The surgeon measures the dimension of bone gap directly on the graduated tines of the wedge opener and selects the plate.

FIGURE 6

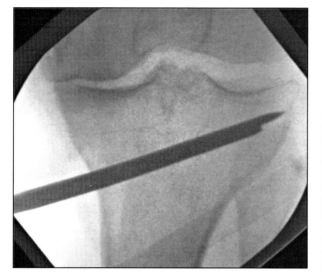

A sharp osteotome, below and parallel to the guide pin, is used to finish the osteotomy, preserving a lateral hinge of about 0.5 cm of intact bone.

Plate Fixation

By removing the handle and, if necessary, one of the wedges, with the other one still in the osteotomy, the plate is easily positioned on the medial cortex of the tibia with the spacer tooth introduced into the osteotomic line. Before fixing the plate, fluoroscopy is used to check the mechanical axis by means of the special guide rod, long enough to extend from the center of the femoral head through the knee to the center of the ankle. When the rod crosses the knee at a lateral point about two thirds (63%) of the tibia plateau, then the angular correction corresponds to the 10° of anatomic valgus that had been planned in advance. However, if the correction is under- or oversized, the plate can be exchanged with one that has a thicker or thinner tooth as needed. The plate is then fixed proximally with two 6.5-mm cancellous screws and distally with two 4.5-mm cortical screws (Figure 8). In the valgus knee, the medial side is the convex side so that the plate can act as a tension band device, conforming to an important biomechanical principle for the effectiveness of the internal fixation.

Bone Grafting

With a skin incision extending from the anterosuperior iliac spine 8 to 10 cm above the iliac crest, two or three corticocancellous bone grafts with the same wedge shape

FIGURE 7

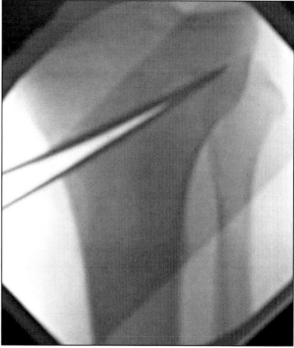

The osteotomy is easily opened with the help of the jack.

FIGURE 8

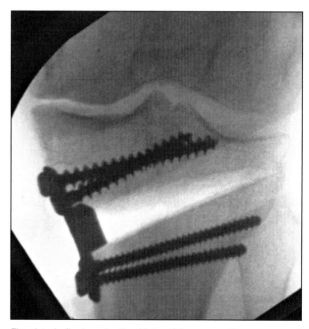

The plate is fixed proximally with two 6.5-mm cancellous screws and distally with two 4.5-mm cortical screws.

FIGURE 9

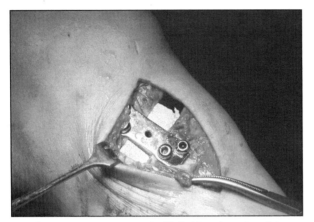

After fixation, the osteotomy gap is filled with wedges of ready to use bone substitute that are available in different sizes (Hatric; Arthrex, Inc, Naples, FL).

FIGURE 11

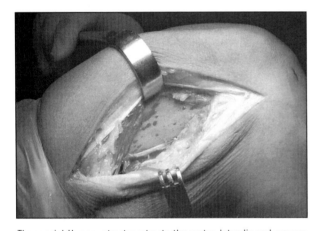

The special Homan retractor retracts the vastus lateralis and exposes the lateral cortex of the femur.

as the osteotomy are obtained; the larger one measures the full correction, while the others are proportionately smaller. The grafts are press-fit to fill the defect. It is also possible to use different grafts, such as bone from the bank or synthetic Hatric (Arthrex, Inc, Naples, FL) (Figure 9) or bovine freeze-dried bone or, according to other authors, no grafts at all. The correct position of the plate and grafts is confirmed with AP and lateral radiographs (Figure 10). One or two drains (the second intra-articular if needed) are prepared, and the wound is closed in a routine manner.

FIGURE 10

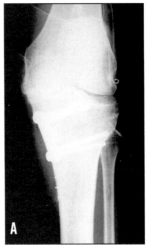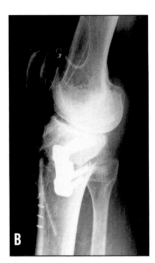

The correct position of the plate and grafts is confirmed with AP (A) and lateral (B) radiographs.

SURGICAL TECHNIQUE OF FEMORAL OSTEOTOMY

Patient Position and Arthroscopy

Positioning and preparation of the patient for femoral osteotomy is the same as for the tibial procedure. The rationale for arthroscopy is the same and is performed with the same intentions as the tibial procedure.

Incision and Exposure

The lateral aspect of the femur is exposed with a standard straight incision through the skin and the fascia starting two fingersbreadth distal to the epicondyle and extending about 12 cm proximally. The dissection is carried down to the vastus lateralis, which is retracted from the posterolateral intermuscular septum by the special dedicated Homan retractor placed ventrally. Perforating vessels should be controlled with ligature or electrocautery. The joint capsule is left intact. The lateral cortex is now exposed. The procedure is facilitated by flexion of the knee (Figure 11).

Osteotomy

The preferred method consists of drilling the Steinmann guide pin into the femur by the free hand; however, the Osteotomy Guide Assembly and the Osteotomy Cutting Guide may be helpful in the proper positioning of the Steinmann guide pin and use of the oscillating saw.

FIGURE 12

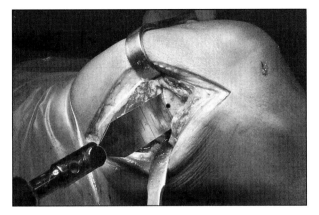

The osteotome must be kept safely parallel and proximal to the guide pin to prevent an intra-articular fracture.

FIGURE 13

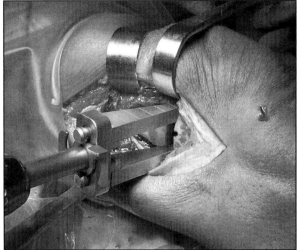

The "wedge opener" is introduced and slowly advanced into the osteotomy.

After perfect positioning of the Steinmann guide pin in a slightly oblique direction (about 20°) from a proximal point on the lateral cortex, three fingersbreadth above the epicondyle and safely off from the trochlear groove to a distal point on the medial cortex, a second Homan retractor is placed dorsally to avoid soft-tissue damage. The osteotomy is started with the power saw just to cut the cortical bone. It is very important to carry out the osteotomy with the blade, the saw, and then the osteotome parallel and proximal to the Steinmann guide pin to help prevent intra-articular fracture (Figure 12). The osteotomy must be perpendicular to the long axis of the femur so that the "T" plate is well oriented with the femoral shaft. After cutting the first few centimeters with the saw, a sharp, flexible, thin osteotome is introduced and driven in all directions into the femur to separate the cancellous bone and the anterior and posterior cortices, ending the osteotomy 0.5 cm before the medial cortex to preserve a hinge of intact bone.

Wedge Opening

After the distraction by the jack, the opener is introduced and slowly advanced until the osteotomy has been opened to obtain the planned realignment of the knee (Figure 13) and the handle is removed. The surgeon measures the dimension of bone gap directly on the graduated wedges of the opener and selects the plate.

Plate Fixation

By removing the handle of the opener, the plate is easily positioned on the lateral cortex of the femur with the spacer tooth introduced into the osteotomic line. If the plate does not fit the femur cortex properly, it must be precontoured by modeling with the bending pliers. Before fixing the plate, we calculate the mechanical axis by means of a special guide rod, long enough to extend from the center of the femoral head to the center of the ankle. This is then checked under fluoroscopy at the passage on the knee joint at approximately the center of the tibial spine for neutral mechanical axis. When the correction is under- or oversized, a different plate with a thicker or thinner tooth is chosen as needed. The plate is then fixed with four cortical screws proximal to the osteotomy and two cancellous screws distally (Figure 14). A lateral plate rather than a medial one is recommended for an important biomechanical reason. When a normal knee with a valgus femorotibial angle is loaded in single-leg stance, the lateral femur is the tension side secondary to the extrinsic varus component of the body weight. In severe genu valgum, the mechanical axis moves laterally and, therefore, the convex medial side is subjected to tensile forces. After osteotomy, the mechanical axis is again moved medially, which returns the tension side of the knee to the lateral side. To act as a tension band, the plate must be applied to the lateral femur. Application of the plate to the medial femur after the osteotomy, as in the closing wedge osteotomy with the AO 90° angled blade plate, violates this principle and may result in a high incidence of failure.

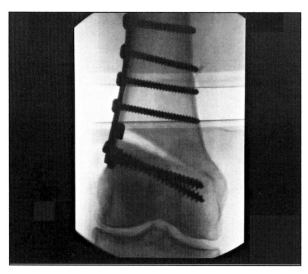

FIGURE 14

The plate is secured to the femur with four cortical screws proximal to the osteotomy and two cancellous screws distally.

FIGURE 16

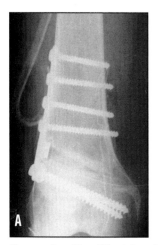
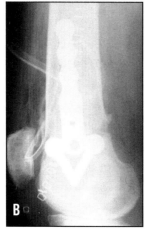

The correct position of the plate and grafts is confirmed with AP (A) and lateral (B) radiographs.

Bone Grafting

The osteotomic defect is normally filled with grafts of autologous bone (Figure 15), or in rarer circumstances, with synthetic bone substitute. In all opening wedge osteotomies that are greater than 7.5 mm, bone grafting is recommended to prevent delayed or nonunion and/or fixation failure. In osteotomies that are 7.5 mm or smaller, the decision to bone graft should be individualized. The

FIGURE 15

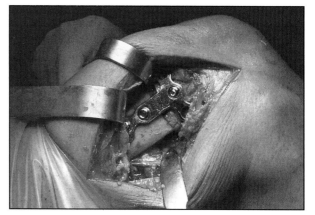

The bone defect normally is filled with grafts of autologous bone.

correct position of the plate and grafts is confirmed with AP and lateral radiographs (Figure 16). One of two drains (one intra-articular) is prepared and the wound is routinely closed.

TECHNICAL PITFALLS AND COMPLICATIONS

The risk of intra-articular fracture is always present. Intra-articular fractures in these patients are more often the result of incorrect positioning of the Steinmann guide pin too close to the joint, leaving a very poor metaphyseal bone stock between the osteotomy and the articular surface. It can also be the result of imperfect finishing of the osteotomy without complete interruption of the anterior, or, more often, posterior cortices, which produces an articular fracture at the moment the knee is stressed in valgus or varus. The osteotomy jack greatly reduces but does not eliminate this risk. Although not easy, in most instances it is possible to repair the fracture with the proximal screws in the tibia, or the distal ones in the femur, introduced, as usual, through the plate.

When the hinge of intact bone is fractured, the osteotomy dislocates. When inspecting the fixation and the alignment of the bone under fluoroscopy, the osteotomy angle may appear subluxated because the tibia, distal to the osteotomy, or the femur, proximal to the osteotomy, dislocates laterally or medially, respectively. Preventing this problem starts with ensuring proper selection of the site for the osteotomy cut. The cut should be proximal enough in the tibia (or distal enough in the femur), to avoid the maximum step-off of the bone profile, thereby ensuring a more stable fixation. An intact bone hinge is essential for stability, and when correctly preserved, it prevents the osteotomy from any possible dislocation. However, if undesired subluxation has occurred despite these precautions, one solution is to fix the corner of the osteotomy with a metallic staple inserted though a contralateral incision.

Failure of the hardware, especially the plates, should be a very rare event. However, a screw can break when weight bearing is allowed too soon postoperatively. Screw breaks also can be caused by a technical error. Imperfect congruence of the tooth plate into the osteotomic space overloads the screws with a lever arm that cannot be resisted. An intact hinge maintains a sort of intrinsic elasticity and, acting as a spring, closes the osteotomy on the tooth, making the fit between the system plate and bone congruent and tight. Conversely, a fissured hinge fails to exert this elastic compression on the opposite side of the bone. The plate may be loose into the bone and the spacer tooth not in contact with both cortices. The screws are designed to support part of the effort to prevent the osteotomy collapse until the bone heals, but they may break because of a fatigue fracture of the metal before complete recovery.

The lateral positioning of the "T" plate also is critical. The osteotomy has to be perfectly oriented in the sagittal plane, perpendicular to the longitudinal axis of the femur to ensure that the long arm of the plate is lying completely on the bone, just in the center of the diaphysis. In fact, the spacer tooth forms a right angle with the plate, which prevents the correct positioning of the long arm on the bone when the osteotomy is oblique with the femur. If the vertical arm is not parallel to the diaphysis, the last upper holes of the plate fall out of the bone, anteriorly or posteriorly to the cortex, making it very difficult to properly fix all of the screws (Figure 17).

Injuries to the vessels are not frequent. The literature reports accidental tears to the anterior tibial artery but only when an extensive lateral approach to the tibia is performed. Tears to the posterior vessels can be safely prevented by correct use of the posterior Homan retractor and maintaining the knee in flexion during surgery.

Thrombophlebitis and infections are complications common to all the other surgical procedures about the inferior limb.

Delayed union may occur, but most osteotomies will result in union with time and partially assisted early weight bearing. Nonunion is also a possibility. In our series

FIGURE 17

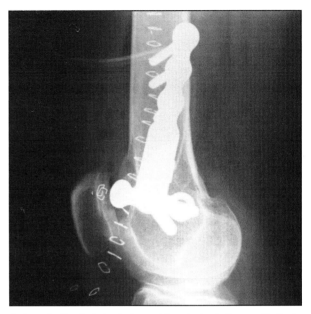

An imperfectly oriented osteotomy, oblique instead of perpendicular to the axis of the femur, leads to a malposition of the vertical arm of the "T" plate.

(43 tibial and 21 femoral osteotomies), there were no nonunions; however, this may depend on the systematic use of the bone grafts to fill the osteotomy.

Peroneal palsy is always a potential complication of tibial valgus closing wedge osteotomy; we have never seen this complication in the opening wedge technique. However, in severe valgus deformities when distal varus osteotomy is performed, a transitory peroneal neurapraxia can occur because of the overstretching of the nerve because of the correction.

It may be incorrect to consider loss of the desired correction as a true complication. In an opening wedge osteotomy, the bone collapse of the grafts might result in a decrease of the angular correction, but the new plates have been shown to be effective in preventing this problem. However, chronic degenerative changes and a high adduction moment contribute to a gradual loss of correction over time.

POSTOPERATIVE MANAGEMENT AND REHABILITATION

Following surgery, the knee is immobilized in a brace in full extension or at slight flexion of about 10° that allows a full range of motion when unlocked. Passive flexion and extension in a continuous passive motion device are started the day after surgery. The drains are removed after 48 hours. Patients are allowed to walk on the second postoperative day with no weight bearing on the affected limb, and they are discharged from the hospital in 4 to 5 days.

When postoperative knee pain and effusion have minimized, restoring normal range of motion in the leg and musculotendinous extensibility (with consideration for biarticular muscles) is fundamental to implementing an exercise program. The program should integrate the trunk, hip, and ankle muscles into dynamic knee stabilization challenges while addressing isolated quadriceps deficiencies. Physical therapy requires continual attention to the balance of protection and function. Although progressive weight bearing and range-of-motion exercises are vital to recovery, early excessive joint loading and terminal knee flexion-extension with external loads can compromise the integrity of the surgical realignment.

Usually within the first 4 weeks, patients are able to completely flex the knee. After 4 weeks (6 in femoral osteotomy), functional weight bearing is allowed. Full weight bearing is normally possible after 6 to 7 weeks (8 or 9 in femoral osteotomy) when the radiographs show satisfactory healing of the bone. Greater emphasis is then placed on restoring normal proprioception and kinesthesia in the involved leg.

While the rehabilitation program progresses to address both anaerobic and aerobic energy systems, increasing fatigue resistance, as evidenced by prolonged maintenance of appropriate body control during functional exercises without apparent discomfort or movement-avoidance patterns, assures the therapist that neuromuscular control for dynamic knee stabilization is improving. Delayed progression may be needed for older patients, particularly if they have not been active recently, and rehabilitation should emphasize active range of motion to facilitate articular cartilage nourishment and preservation.

ALTERNATIVE SURGICAL TECHNIQUES

Once the principle of the angular correction is well accepted as an effective treatment of knee OA that is associated with varus or valgus deformity, the osteotomy has to be considered a valid therapeutic modality above all the techniques proposed in the literature.

The original closing wedge osteotomies were followed some years later by opening wedge osteotomies after Coventry[1] described his technique of high tibial osteotomy. From the perspective of correction, the same results can be achieved in modifying the limb alignment by adding or subtracting a wedge from the tibia or the femur, on the condition that the addition or subtraction is on the opposite side of the bone. We currently prefer a medial opening wedge osteotomy of the tibia to correct a varus knee. However, the closing wedge osteotomy is a good alternative, and many authors, including ourselves until 1992, can obtain the same results with a lateral closing wedge osteotomy.

Closing wedge tibial osteotomy in the varus knee is performed through a lateral access with a curvilinear incision along the lateral tibial crest extending above the fibular head. The tibiofibular joint is identified and disrupted with an osteotome, or the fibular shaft is interrupted at the level of the neck or distally, in a safer area, with a second incision. Two Steinmann guide pins are drilled into the tibial metaphysis to delineate the sides of a triangular wedge of bone, which has to be removed. Pin placement is critical because the precision of the osteotomy depends on it. Many of the complications, such as an intra-articular fracture, can be avoided with this technique. Many guide systems are available to optimize the placement of the pins, and coordinate-cutting jigs facilitate management of the oscillating saw during the operation; however, many authors prefer a free hand technique under fluoroscopy. Using the pins as guides, the blade, oscillating saw, and the osteotome resect a bone wedge to be removed from the metaphysis. The surgeon then "closes" the tibia to attain the correction. Other options to repair the osteotomy are available from the classic lateral buttress plate to the special staples, which are stepped to better fit the bone step on the lateral cortex created by the osteotomy, to the external fixator. The closing wedge technique is based on an intact hinge of cortical bone on the opposite side.

There are many intraoperative concerns and pitfalls. Protection of the peroneal nerve is necessary during the procedure. The osteotomy should be performed slowly to allow the medial hinge to remain intact. The osteotomy should be away from the joint line, under the guide pin, to prevent inadvertent fracture of the tibial plateau. Sizing the wedge to attain a precise correction is much more difficult with the closing wedge technique than it is with the opening wedge technique because of the two cuts instead of only one. The position of the blade relative to the two pins, either under the proximal and above the distal pin or under the pins for both the bone cuts, significantly influences the size of the wedge, which is always smaller when the oscillating saw cuts the bone at the inner sides of the pins.

Following the closing wedge technique, there is an advantageous variation of the rehabilitation protocol. Depending on the reliability of the fixation, patients usually can anticipate weight bearing and, starting from the very early postoperative days, are able to walk without assistance of crutches or a cane within the first month.

Various authors have recommended other tibial osteotomy procedures for specific situations. One procedure is the barrel-vault osteotomy, which has the advantage of not significantly altering leg length; another is the Maquet osteotomy, which allows anterior tubercle translation when associated with patellofemoral symptoms. Each of these procedures is somewhat more complex and difficult than the previously described techniques and should be left to surgeons experienced in these settings.

The distal femoral osteotomy is sometimes preferred to the closing wedge technique. A longitudinal incision is made over the medial femoral condyle extending proximally. The osteotomy is then performed in the supracondylar region of the femur under fluoroscopic control. The fixation device, a 90° condylar blade plate, is placed with the blade located distally to the osteotomic line. A wedge of bone is then removed to allow the plate to rest snugly against the cortex, correcting the deformity by impacting the proximal fragment into the distal supracondylar region, where a step-off is expected. The precise degree of correction here depends greatly on preoperative planning and is less influenced by the one or two cuts technique because the correction is strictly related to the impaction of the fragments, one into the other, instead of the dimension of the wedge removed as in the tibial closing wedge technique. The procedure requires an intimate knowledge of the fixation device to avoid the most common complications that include fixation failure and late fracture of the blade plate. After the plate has been secured to the shaft of the femur with a standard technique, the bone wedge is used to graft the area about the step-off.

In the mild valgus deformities of the knee, Chambat and associates[6] propose a tibial closing wedge technique. As previously explained, the obliquity of the joint line can be a serious problem in the varus correction of a valgus deformity; the normal solution to this problem is to perform the correction proximally to the joint in the supra-

condylar region of the femur. But when the deformity measures less than 10° of valgus, a limited tibial correction is possible without invalidating the final result because of an exaggerated tilting of the joint line. The advantage of this technique is a full correction of the valgus malalignment, not only in knee extension but also when the knee is flexed, whereas the supracondylar osteotomy cannot influence the deformity in flexion because the realignment is limited to the distal femoral condyles and leaves the deformity of the posterior condyles unchanged.

RESULTS

In the international literature, many series have shown encouraging middle-term results following high tibial osteotomy. Most authors agree that there is a gradual decline in the quality of the result with time. In general, the high tibial osteotomy has been shown to be effective for approximately 5 years in up to 90% of the patients and for over 10 years in about two thirds (about 65%).

In a review of 139 knees following high tibial osteotomy, Aglietti and associates[7] noted good to excellent results in 64% of knees after a follow-up period of at least 10 years. The authors concluded that high tibial osteotomy is a reliable method for relieving pain in the varus osteoarthritic knee. However, a tendency for results to deteriorate with time was observed; 64% had satisfactory results with more than 10 years' follow-up, 70% with 6 to 10 years, and 87% with 2 to 5 years.

Insall and associates[3] reported good results in 97% of patients at 2 years, 85% at 5 years, and 63% at 9 years. At 9 years, only 37% of these patients were pain-free. Deterioration in these patients is primarily the result of time and not recurrence, but in contrast with Insall and associates, Aglietti and associates[7] reported that deterioration of outcomes is the result of recurrence.

Müller and associates[8] used elastic high tibial valgus osteotomy in a series of 100 consecutive patients with grade III and IV OA between 1989 and 1990. At 3 to 4 years' follow-up, they reported the following results. Correction angle (minimum 4°, maximum 18°): for preoperative relative varus, average 7.1°; for effective correction, 8.9°; and for postoperative femorotibial, 183°. Patient subjective evaluation: 26% very satisfied, 52% satisfied, 18% partially satisfied, 8% not satisfied.

From our personal experience we can present a series of 43 patients, using the opening wedge technique with an average follow-up of 7 years (Figure 13). The average age was 49 years; 25 were men and 18 women. The results were evaluated according to both the International Knee Documentation Committee (IKDC) rating scale and the Hospital for Special Surgery (HSS) score system as follows.

Before the osteotomies, 17 patients belonged to group "C" and 26 to group "D" of the IKDC rating scale; of the patients considered 6 to 8 years after surgery, 23 were passed to group "B" and 20 to group "C." All the patients have improved by at least one category.

The same patients evaluated with the HSS score system resulted in 7 good, 24 fair, and 12 poor knees before the osteotomies; postoperative results were 16 excellent, 22 good, and 5 fair. These particularly satisfying results probably resulted from our incorrect use of the HSS scoring system, which was intended for the evaluation of results in prosthetic replacement surgery.

The results of distal femur osteotomy are satisfying, especially when considered, again, as a midterm evaluation.

In a study of 21 knees, Finkelstein and associates[9] reported 64% of survival after 10 years. This analysis demonstrated that the results of the supracondylar osteotomy were similar to those of the high tibial osteotomy performed for the treatment of medial compartment OA.

In 1988, Healy and associates[10] reported a series of 23 varus femoral osteotomies with 4 years follow-up. The results were evaluated according to the HSS score. After surgery, the knees improved from an average 65 points preoperative score to a score of 86, and 86% of patients expressed satisfaction with the outcome.

In 1990, Miniaci and associates[11] reported 86% good and excellent results in a series of 40 femoral osteotomies with a follow-up of 5.5 years.

From our personal experience, we can present a series of 21 patients operated on with the opening wedge technique, with a follow-up of 6.5 years. The average age was 43 years; 9 were men and 12 women. The results were evaluated according to both the IKDC rating scale and HSS score system as follows.

Before the osteotomies, eight patients belonged to group "C" and 13 to group "D" of the IKDC rating scale; the patients were then considered 5 to 7 years after surgery. Twelve were passed to group "B" and 9 to group "C." All of the patients improved by at least one category.

The same cases evaluated with the HSS score system resulted in 14 fair and 7 poor knees before the osteotomies; postoperative results were 11 excellent and 10 good.

REFERENCES

1. Coventry MB: Osteotomy about the knee for degenerative and rheumatoid arthritis. *J Bone Joint Surg Am* 1973;55:23-48.

2. Insall JN, Shoji H, Mayer V: High tibial osteotomy: A five year evaluation. *J Bone Joint Surg Am* 1974;56:1397-1405.

3. Insall JN, Joseph DM, Msika C: High tibial osteotomy for varus gonarthrosis. *J Bone Joint Surg Am* 1984;66:1040-1048.

4. Dugdale TW, Noyes FR, Styer D: Preoperative planning for high tibial osteotomy: The effect of lateral tibiofemoral separation and tibiofemoral length. *Clin Orthop* 1992;274:248-264.

5. Rosenberg TD, Paulos LE, Parker RD, et al: The forty-five-degree posteroanterior weight-bearing radiograph of the knee. *J Bone Joint Surg Am* 1988;70:1479-1483.

6. Chambat P, Ait Si Selmi T, Dejour D, et al: Varus tibial osteotomy. *Oper Tech Sports Med* 2000;1:44-47.

7. Aglietti P, Rinonapoli E, Stringa G, et al: Tibial osteotomy for the varus osteoarthritic knee. *Clin Orthop* 1983;176:239-251.

8. Müller W, Kentsch A, Schafer N: The elastic high tibia valgus osteotomy in the varus deformity. *Oper Tech Sports Med* 2000;1:19-26.

9. Finkelstein JA, Gross AE, Davis A: Varus osteotomy of the distal part of the femur: A survivorship analysis. *J Bone Joint Surg Am* 1996;78:1348-1352.

10. Healy WL, Anglen JO, Wasilewski, SA, Krackow KA: Distal femoral varus osteotomy. *J Bone Joint Surg Am* 1988;70:102-109.

11. Miniaci A, Grossmann SP, Jakob RP: Supracondylar femoral varus osteotomy in the treatment of valgus knee deformity. *Am J Knee Surg* 1990;2:65-73.

CHAPTER 4

MENISCUS TRANSPLANTATION: INDICATIONS AND FOLLOW-UP

RENÉ VERDONK, MD, PhD
FREDRIK ALMQUIST, MD, PhD

On November 16, 1883, Thomas Annandale[1] was the first surgeon to perform a medial meniscal suture. The anterior horn of a medial meniscus that had been torn 10 months previously was sutured to its former peripheral attachment. The patient was discharged after 10 weeks with an almost normally functioning knee.

Since that time, arthrotomy and meniscectomy have become common orthopaedic procedures. In the 1950s and the 1960s, total meniscectomy was performed for almost any meniscal tear that was diagnosed on clinical examination. In the last two decades, however, arthroscopy of the knee joint has provided surgeons with a means of performing adequate meniscectomy following the technical rules laid down by several authors, including Jackson,[2] Sprague,[3] and Rand.[4] The period between 1970 and 1980 showed that with a carefully executed arthroscopic meniscectomy for a torn medial meniscus, function was restored in more than 90% of patients.

The short-term results of these resections are comparable to those of open meniscectomy with regard to the medial compartment of the knee. In the longer term and in the event of medial meniscectomy, factors such as varus malalignment and mechanical overload increase the risk of degeneration of the load-bearing cartilage in the medial compartment (Figure 1). Not only is the buffer function of the semilunar cartilage absent between the femoral condyle and medial tibial plateau, but the stabilizing factor (ie, the meniscal wall) also is lacking. As a result, there is an increased anteroposterior shift of the femoral condyle in relation to the medial tibial plateau (Figure 2).

Any ligamentous laxity produced by the initial trauma increases the degenerative changes in the load-bearing area. Of even more importance but medically uncontrollable is the magnitude of the mechanical load. This load is a separate element dependent on the weight of the patient and on occupational and sports activities.

The same findings apply to older age groups. The short-term results of arthroscopic meniscectomy are superior to those of open total meniscectomy because of the preservation of the meniscal wall. Again, the quality of the load-bearing cartilage will determine the functional outcome in this age group. In the long run, only 50% of patients benefit from arthroscopic medial meniscectomy. These fair to poor results in the older age groups have caused orthopaedic surgeons to be cautious about these negative consequences of meniscectomy; thus, a meniscal suture is performed whenever feasible. Within a short time, the meniscal suture leads to meniscal healing, resulting in a functionally competent knee and anatomic restoration in 90% of patients.[5]

If chondral congruity is indeed improved by the presence of the medial meniscus under loading conditions, then these findings certainly apply to the lateral compartment. The convex lateral femoral condyle articulates with an almost convex lateral tibial plateau. The contact area between both cartilaginous elements is flattened and widened only because of the presence of the O-shaped

FIGURE 1

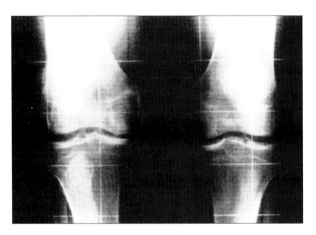

In the event of a medial meniscectomy (right knee), factors such as varus malalignment and mechanical overload increase the risk of degeneration in the load-bearing medial compartment.

lateral meniscus. Greater caution is advised in the treatment of a lateral meniscal lesion; clinical experience has shown that problems may arise even after correct and adequate resection of a torn lateral meniscus.[2-4,6]

ANIMAL STUDIES

In animal studies, meniscal allografts and tendon autografts have been shown to heal to the capsule.[7] They are repopulated with host cells and revascularized. However, neither tendon nor meniscal allografts attain the properties of normal menisci. Even though they appear to offer some protection to the cartilage in the knee joint, no evidence exists that degenerative changes can be prevented. It is not clear whether the cellular repopulation is sufficient to restore adequate biomechanical properties. Tissue-engineered grafts are still under investigation and are showing promising results.

TYPES OF MENISCAL SUBSTITUTES

Meniscal Prostheses

Polytetrafluoroethylene and polyethylene terephthalate prostheses have some chondroprotective effect in the rabbit knee. However, with respect to the biomechanical properties, the implanted joint resembles a meniscectomized joint rather than a normal knee joint. Other types of implants are being investigated.[8]

FIGURE 2

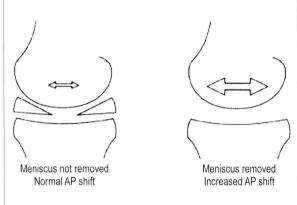

Meniscus not removed
Normal AP shift

Meniscus removed
Increased AP shift

With total meniscectomy, an increased anteroposterior shift is expected.

Scaffolds

Collagen scaffolds have been implanted, serving as a template for the regeneration of meniscal cartilage. Animal experiments have shown that host chondrocytes migrate into the new tissue. Although scaffolds were originally designed for partially meniscectomized joints, their use for complete meniscal replacement remains under investigation.

Fat Pad Autografts

In sheep, the transplanted pediculated infrapatellar fat pad results in the development of a meniscus-like structure within 6 months.[7,9,10] The tissue deteriorates over time, however, as observed at 1 year. It remains weak and is not comparable to the original meniscal tissue.

Tendon Autografts

Disease transmission can be avoided by using autografts from sheep. A patellar tendon graft remodels to meniscus-like tissue.[7,9] After 1 year, strong circumferential collagen fiber bundles can be identified. However, the biomechanical properties seem to be inferior to the original meniscal tissue.

Meniscal Allografts

Numerous animal experiments with this type of implant have been conducted.[7] Results seem to be dependent on the tissue preservation methods. The allografts have been shown to generally heal to the capsule and be revascularized and repopulated with host cells.

FIGURE 3

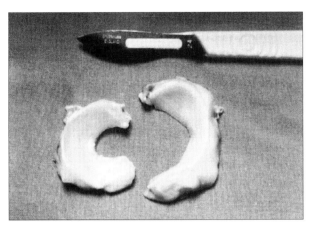

The menisci are removed from the donor knee joint. In this case, only the medial meniscus is suitable for transplantation; the lateral meniscus shows degeneration and cannot be used.

FIGURE 4

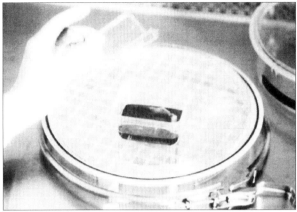

The plastic container is placed in an incubation chamber at a constant temperature of 37°C under continuous airflow.

HUMAN EXPERIENCE

The goals of meniscal replacement are to reduce the pain experienced by some patients following meniscus resection, avoid or reduce the risk of degenerative arthritis following resection, and optimally restore the mechanical properties of the knee joint after resection. The results of meniscus transplantation have been reported in several series of patients who were operated on with different techniques. Controlled studies of meniscus replacement in humans do not exist.

Harvest

Menisci are ideally harvested within 12 hours of the onset of ischemia.[11] In fresh-frozen grafts, few cells survive. Cryopreservation allows the fibrochondrocytes to be preserved in 10% to 30% of samples. Meniscal implants must be readily available for transplantation and free of transmittable diseases. The clinical immune response should be eliminated.

The meniscal bodies are removed from general organ donors and frozen (Figure 3). The grafts are either fresh-frozen to −78°C or frozen using a cryopreservation technique, in which the material is progressively deep frozen to −178°C using dimethylsulfoxide. According to Fabbriciani and associates,[12] the cryopreservation technique does not provide better histologic results after implantation in animals. The fresh-frozen allografts are inexpensive and easy to store.

For the allograft to be viable, donor menisci are removed in an operating room under strict aseptic conditions, after harvesting of other organs from living (multiple-organ donors) or nonheartbeating donors. The cold ischemia time must not exceed 12 hours, which is the amount of time during which the meniscus remains viable. Through a transverse arthrotomy, the lateral collateral and cruciate ligaments are divided and the knee is dislocated anteriorly.

The menisci are transported in a sterile physiologic solution to the tissue bank. Under sterile conditions, the specimens are placed in culture using Dulbecco's modified Eagle's medium with 0.002-M L-glutamine, 1/1,000 antibiotic-antimycotic suspension (streptomycin 10 mg/mL, penicillin 10 U/mL, fungizone 0.025 mg/mL) and 20% of the recipient's serum. This serum is prepared from the recipient's blood by centrifugation.

The menisci are stored in a plastic container to which 70 mL of incubation medium is added. The container is placed in a modular incubation chamber at a constant temperature of 37°C and under continuous airflow (95% air and 5% CO_2)[13] (Figure 4). Humidity is controlled by placing an open receptacle filled with sterile water in the incubation chamber. The incubation media are replaced every 3 days. The recipient's sera are stored at −18°C and are suitable for clinical use for a maximum of 6 weeks following venipuncture.

Under these conditions, transplanted allograft remains

FIGURE 5

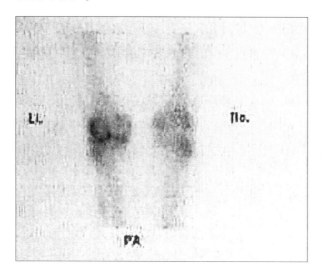

Disruption of homeostasis of the subchondral bone is adequately visualized by a technetium Tc 99m bone scan.

FIGURE 6

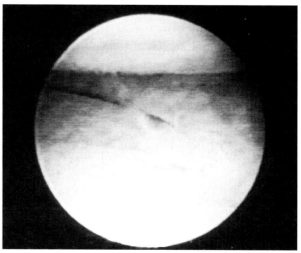

Arthroscopy is the only means to efficiently evaluate the chondral status of the knee and to exclude extensive chondral deterioration (from grade 4).

viable, producing fibrochondrocytes, proteoglycans, and collagen fiber structures.[14] Normal cellular function is expected from the moment of implantation, inducing a potentially normal meniscal function that may prove to be of great advantage when compared with frozen allografts.

Preoperative Planning

Thorough preoperative planning is mandatory to obtain good clinical results with meniscus transplantation.[15] Any pathology, in addition to the missing meniscus, should be identified, including malalignment and ligament instability. The cartilage should be closely evaluated for any changes. It is not known how accurately the donor meniscus needs to match the size of the original meniscus to achieve healing and regeneration.[16]

To properly assess any axial malalignment and joint space narrowing, weight-bearing radiographs are mandatory. Weight-bearing radiographs in 45° of flexion and 10° of ray inclination allow for better visualization of degenerative joint disease. AP views are also essential to exclude any major bone pathology and to identify potential subchondral condensation and cystic degeneration.

Disruption of homeostasis of the subchondral bone is properly visualized with a technetium Tc 99m bone scan (Figure 5). This modality confirms subchondral overload, and it can be used for follow-up purposes. After menis-

cus transplantation, a joint that functions normally may appear normal on a bone scan.

Both the donor's and the recipient's joints can be sized using CT. This technique is used to evaluate the recipient's knee joint, as precise information about size of the allograft is obtained when it is removed from the donor and measured.[16]

MRI is mandatory to illustrate preoperative findings. Indeed, meniscal allografting is indicated only in totally meniscectomized knees. Theoretically, dynamic MRI may provide valuable information about the mechanical behavior of the knee (ie, ligaments, menisci) both preoperatively and postoperatively.

Arthroscopy is the only means by which to evaluate the chondral status of the knee and exclude extensive chondral deterioration (from grade 4) (Figure 6). Arthroscopy also can confirm that the meniscus is actually missing. If arthroscopy has been performed previously, information (photographs or video images) should be made available to the surgeon and correlated with MRI findings.

Surgical Technique

Surgery should be minimally invasive, preserving the original meniscal insertion points.[17] An open technique is preferred for medial transplantation, whereas the arthroscopic approach facilitates lateral implantation.

FIGURE 7

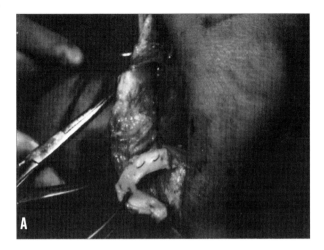
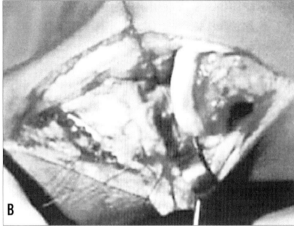

A, The threaded viable meniscal allograft is inserted from posterior to anterior. An osteotomy of the femoral insertion of the lateral collateral ligament facilitates access to the posterolateral corner of the lateral knee joint. **B,** Once the lateral meniscus is in place, fixation of the anterior horn at its original location allows for proper fitting of the meniscus in situ.

General or epidural anesthesia is induced and a tourniquet is applied. The patient is placed supine, and a medial anterior arthrotomy is performed. The anterior third of the medial meniscus is incised just medial of the anterior horn insertion. This anatomically located insertion is used to reattach the meniscal allograft to its original anterior horn, sometimes strengthened with bone anchor fixation.

The potential meniscal remnant, if any, is resected down to the meniscosynovial rim until a bleeding surface is exposed. Care is taken to leave the meniscal wall in situ. This allows the meniscal allograft to be inserted onto the meniscal wall and thus respect the circumferential extrusion forces after implantation. Whether a standard medioposterior incision is made to facilitate transplantation and further removal of the meniscal remnant or a flake osteotomy of the medial collateral ligament is performed, the meniscus is inserted and fixed using No. 2.0 PDS sutures (Ethicon, Ethnor JJ, Neuilly, France). Small needles are required to secure the posterior horn in its anatomic location. If bone plug fixation is required, the technique is more complicated and the risk of improper placement is higher.[18] The medial collateral ligament, with its bony insertion, is replaced at its original location and fixed with staples or a screw and washer.

Because of inherent increased varus laxity versus valgus laxity, an arthroscopic technique is indicated for lateral meniscal transplantation. The lateral meniscal allograft is prepared, either with a separate bone plug or bone rim, or without bone blocks. The allograft is inserted through a lateral arthroscopic portal, allowing tight passage through the skin incision.[19]

In an open approach, an extended lateral skin incision allows for an osteotomy with a bone plug of the lateral collateral ligament and popliteal tendon insertion. This approach opens up the lateral compartment and allows implantation of the lateral meniscus from posterior to anterior (Figure 7). The anterior horn of the lateral meniscus is fixed using bone anchoring at the anatomic location (Figure 8).

Results

Between 1989 and 2002, we implanted 108 viable meniscal allografts in 105 patients (74 male, 31 female). A total of 47 left knees and 61 right knees were treated. Of these, 61% were lateral menisci, 36% were medial, and 3% were bilateral. Follow-up ranged from 11 months to 13.8 years (mean, 7 years).

Twenty-two associated procedures were performed in the study group. In patients with malalignment, a corrective osteotomy was performed. In a few patients, the anterior cruciate ligament (ACL)-deficient knee was treated with an ACL-plasty using tendon allografts.

Complications developed in 12 patients in the postoperative period. Three patients had transient synovitis, and

FIGURE 8

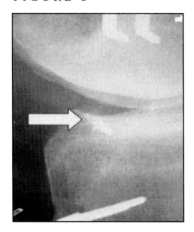

Bone anchors can help stabilize the anterior horn at its anatomic position.

FIGURE 9

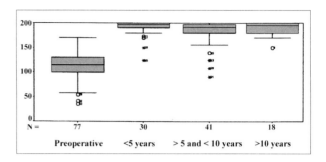

At 10 years, 5 patients had undergone an arthroplasty, 2 died of unrelated causes, and 1 had rheumatoid arthritis. Between 5 and 10 years postoperatively, 9% of the patients underwent a total knee arthroplasty.

three patients required mobilization under anesthesia. These complications occurred only when combined surgery was performed. Two patients had transient superficial infections, and one patient had a transient drop foot in association with a high tibial varus osteotomy. One patient required reinsertion after lateral collateral ligament osteotomy and refixation. In two cases of pseudarthrosis after high tibial osteotomy, reintervention was necessary.

A total of 87 of 105 patients were included in the study (61 male, 26 female). Of the 18 patients who were dropped, 9 underwent total or unicondylar knee arthroplasty because of painful progression of osteoarthritis with severe functional impairment, 4 could be contacted only by telephone, 2 died of causes not related to surgery, 2 were lost to follow-up, and 1 had rheumatoid arthritis.

Eighty-seven percent of patients reported that they would undergo the same surgery if required. Only 38% of the patients returned to their former occupation, whereas 62% returned to a more sedentary type of work.

In the clinical evaluation, patients were scored using the Hospital for Special Surgery (HSS) score. The mean score of all patients was 185 points postoperatively. A score of 175 was arbitrarily chosen as a good to excellent result. A total of 83% of patients scored higher than 175, 16% scored between 100 and 175, and only 1% (1 patient) scored less than 100. The pain score increased significantly from 13.6 preoperatively to 43.2 postoperatively ($P < 0.05$). No significant statistical difference in HSS score was found, neither between medial and lateral meniscal transplants ($P = 0.17$) nor between medial transplants with and without high tibial osteotomy. In the subgroup, we

did not find any difference in pain relief. The HSS score increased postoperatively and remained fairly constant afterward. At 10 years postoperatively, 35.7% of all patients were lost to follow-up. Of these, five had undergone an arthroplasty, two had died of causes not related to knee surgery, and one was diagnosed with rheumatoid arthritis. Between 5 and 10 years postoperatively, 9% of patients had undergone a total knee arthroplasty (Figure 9).

Wirth and associates[20-22] reported comparable results with deep frozen meniscal implants. When lyophilization techniques are used for meniscal preservation, less than optimal results are obtained.

Rehabilitation

Some authors recommend continuous passive motion during the first postoperative days.[9] Passive and active non–weight-bearing motion from 0° to 60° or 90° is advised for 4 to 6 weeks. It is generally recommended that weight bearing in the first 4 to 6 weeks should be brace controlled with full extension to avoid shear forces on the allograft. These restrictions arise from basic knowledge of the meniscal loading pattern during motion. Load stress on the meniscus increases with increased knee flexion; in particular, the medial posterior horn is stressed at knee angles exceeding 60°, but femoral anterior-posterior translation and rotation also affect the load pattern of the meniscus. However, some weight bearing should be allowed, as controlled stress stimulates collagen synthesis and increases the strength of connective tissues (Wolff's law). Consequently, the meniscal allograft probably also benefits from repetitive hoop stress during knee joint

FIGURE 10

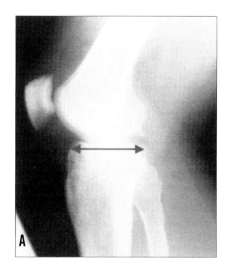 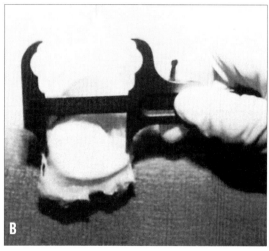

Radiographic sizing is used in the planning of meniscal transplant surgery in a clinical setting.

loading and adapts with increased tensile properties over time. However, these changes occur only if the repopulated host cells in the graft are sufficient to restore the meniscal collagen architecture and strength. These rather crucial questions in meniscal allograft transplantation remain unanswered and should be addressed in biomechanical studies.

Approximately 6 weeks postoperatively, gait training and loaded, closed-chain activities up to 90° flexion can be initiated. Among other beneficial effects, this training stimulates knee proprioception. Muscle strength training is also important in rehabilitation, particularly quadriceps strength because this muscle serves as a secondary shock absorber to the knee joint and relieves load stress on the meniscus. From 6 to 12 months, full weight bearing, full range of motion, and return to previous activities are recommended.

DISCUSSION

Several issues still stand in meniscal allograft transplantation. Its aim is to relieve pain in meniscectomized knee joints but also to avoid further degenerative osteoarthritis. Furthermore, fixation of the meniscus in the clinical setting remains an issue: should bone blocks be used in medial meniscal transplantation or a bone bridge used in lateral meniscal transplantation? Several in vitro studies have shown that horn fixation with bone blocks or bridge of the meniscal transplant is recommended to withstand the hoop stresses on the meniscal bodies when weight

bearing is initiated postoperatively. However, reconstructing the original and anatomic insertion of the former meniscus can be difficult. Lazovic and associates[23] and Aagaard[10] have shown that with incongruent transplant fixation, the transplant biomechanics are worse than when total meniscectomy is performed in laboratory animals.

Optimal insertion of the meniscal horns with bone blocks is tedious, if not impossible, and the level of the implant with respect to the joint line is of major importance. Both the meniscal plugs in the medial transplants and the bone bridge in the lateral transplants need to be drilled properly with regard to location and depth so as to allow the transplant to sit flat on the tibial surface. In open knee surgery, the depth of the plugs can be readily evaluated and adjusted if necessary. In arthroscopic-assisted implantation, this is a complicated and time-consuming procedure.

Proper preoperative sizing of the meniscus is done using radiographic measurements (Figure 10). McDermott and associates[16] described the complexity and variability of the meniscal body, not only in length and width but also in height. Consequently, the ideal transplant shape depends on highly individual factors and, hence, is almost nonexistent. Not using bone blocks would allow for more appropriate stretching and molding of the meniscal transplant, thereby allowing a better clinical fit.

In almost all instances of total meniscectomy, both the anterior and the posterior horns of the former meniscus have been preserved. Thus, the anterior and posterior horns of the transplant can be securely fixed to these struc-

FIGURE 11

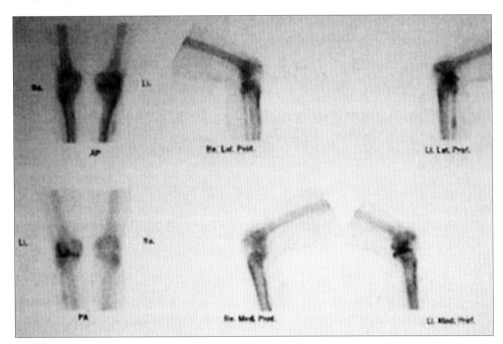

Even at 2 years' follow-up, a technetium Tc 99m bone scan of a left lateral meniscal transplant is still abnormal.

tures. In most meniscectomized knees, the meniscal rim is still present. It is our conviction that this rim serves as a strong envelope, encapsulating the knee compartment. By firm fixation of the meniscal horns and secure suturing to the rim, the meniscus transplant transmits loads under axial compression and is therefore functional.[18,23,24] In our recent unpublished study comparing transplanted lateral menisci to normal menisci in vivo using MRI and ultrasound, the transplanted lateral meniscus was found to partially extrude from the knee joint. The anterior horn of the transplanted lateral meniscus extruded more than the posterior horn. Under axial load, however, the transplanted lateral meniscus did not show more extrusion than the meniscus in the nonloaded situation. The same stable behavior was noted for the normal lateral meniscus. The authors concluded that the transplanted lateral meniscus, with firm fixation of the horns and sutured to the rim, is capable of transmitting loads under axial compression.

SUMMARY AND CONCLUSIONS

The general clinical indication for meniscal transplantation is disabling pain after total meniscectomy in a skeletally mature individual. The healing of the graft to the capsule is apparent on follow-up arthroscopy. Revascularization and cell repopulation have been observed but to a variable degree. In routine clinical practice, lateral meniscectomized knee joints more often appear to be an indication for surgery than knees in which the medial meniscus has been resected because valuable alternatives exist to alleviate medial compartmental knee pain. Combined concomitant surgery can influence the appreciation of the result.

Graft preservation does not lead to variable clinical results. Frozen or cryopreserved allografts appear to offer the most promising short-term results. Viable meniscal allografts appear to survive transplantation as donor fibrochondrocytes are found on a DNA fingerprinting evaluation at 2 years. The clinical outcome does not correlate with meniscal imaging.

No clinical proof exists that substitutes can protect the hyaline cartilage of the femur and tibia in the case of meniscal substitution. It is unclear whether normal homeostasis can be obtained in the long-term (Figure 11). Three factors, however, have been found to impair meniscal substitute function: poor fixation at the anterior and posterior meniscal horn; limited contact of the transplant with the articulating surfaces of the knee; and abnormal horn positioning.

ACKNOWLEDGMENTS

The authors thank Bart Claus, Alex Demurie, Carl De Meulemeester, Patrick De Smet, Can Hürel, Tom Lootens, Franky Steenbrugge, Peter Vandaele, Koen Van Den Abbeele, Peter Verdonk, and Patricia Verstraete for their valuable contributions. Also special acknowledgments to Monique De Pauw for her secretarial work and assistance in the preparation of the manuscript and to Iris Wojtowicz for the English revision of the text.

REFERENCES

1. Annandale TH: An operation for displaced semilunar cartilage. *BMJ* 1885;1:779-781.

2. Jackson RW: The role of arthroscopy in the management of the arthritic knee. *Clin Orthop* 1974;101:28-35.

3. Sprague NF III: Arthroscopic debridement for degenerative knee joint disease. *Clin Orthop* 1981;160:118-123.

4. Rand JA: Arthroscopic management of degenerative meniscus tears in patients with degenerative arthritis. *Arthroscopy* 1985;1:253-258.

5. De Meulemeester C, Verdonk R, Van Eetvelde G, Claessens H: The value of CT scan in the evaluation of meniscal sutures. *Proceedings of the 103rd Annual Meeting of the American Orthopaedic Association.* Boston, Massachusetts, 1990, p 103.

6. Aagaard H, Verdonk R: Function of the normal meniscus and consequences of meniscal resection. *Scand J Med Sci Sports* 1999;9:134-140.

7. Kohn D, Verdonk R, Aagaard H, Seil R, Dienst M: Meniscal substitutes: Animal experience. *Scand J Med Sci Sports* 1999;9:141-145.

8. Messner K, Kohn D, Verdonk R: Future research in meniscal replacement. *Scand J Med Sci Sports* 1999;9:181-183.

9. Kohn D, Aagaard H, Verdonk R, Dienst M, Seil S: Postoperative follow-up and rehabilitation after meniscus replacement. *Scand J Med Sci Sports* 1999;9:177-180.

10. Aagaard H: Meniscal allograft transplantation in sheep. University of Kopenhagen, Copenhagen, Amsterdam, 1998. Thesis.

11. Verdonk R, Kohn D: Harvest and conservation of meniscal allografts. *Scand J Med Sci Sports* 1999;9:158-159.

12. Fabbriciani C, Lucania L, Milano G, Schiavone PA, Evangelisti M: Meniscal allografts: Cryopreservation vs deep-frozen technique. An experimental study in goats. *Knee Surg Sports Traum Arthrosc* 1997;5:124-134.

13. Verbruggen G, Verdonk R, Veys EM, et al: Human meniscal proteoglycan metabolism in long-term tissue culture. *Knee Surg Sports Traumatol Arthrosc* 1996;4:57-63.

14. Verdonk R: Viable meniscal allografts. Ghent University, Ghent, Belgium, 1992. Thesis.

15. Verdonk R, Kohn D: Meniscus transplantation: Preoperative planning. *Scand J Med Sci Sports* 1999;9:160-161.

16. McDermott ID, Sharifi F, Bull AM, Gupte CM, Thomas RW, Amis AA: An anatomical study of meniscal allograft sizing. *Knee Surg Sports Traumatol Arthrosc* 2003 (epub ahead of print).

17. Goble EM, Verdonk R, Kohn D: Arthroscopic and open surgical techniques for meniscus replacement: Meniscal allograft transplantation and tendon autograft transplantation. *Scand J Med Sci Sports* 1999;9:168-176.

18. Messner K, Verdonk R: Is it necessary to anchor the meniscal transplants with bone plugs? A mini-battle. *Scand J Med Sci Sports* 1999;9:186-187.

19. Yoldas EA, Sekiya JK, Irrgang JJ, Fu FH, Harner CD: Arthroscopically assisted meniscal allograft transplantation with and without combined anterior cruciate ligament reconstruction. *Knee Surg Sports Traumatol Arthrosc* 2003 (epub ahead of print).

20. Wirth CJ, Milachowski KA, Weismeier K: Die Meniskustransplantation im Tierexperiment und erste klinische Ergebnisse. *Z Orthop* 1986;124:508-512.

21. Wirth CJ, Peter G, Milachowski KA, Weismeier KG: Long-term results of meniscal allograft transplantation. *Am J Sports Med* 2002;30:174-181.

22. Peters G, Wirth CJ: The current state of meniscal allograft transplantation and replacement. *Knee* 2003;10:19-31.

23. Lazovic D, Wirth CJ, Knösel T, Gossé M, Maschek HG: Meniscus replacement using incongruent transplants: An experimental study. *Z Orthop Ihre Grenzgeb* 1997;135:131-137.

24. Chen MI, Branch TP, Hutton WC: Is it important to secure the horns during lateral meniscal transplantation? A cadaveric study. *Arthroscopy* 1996;12:174-181.

CHAPTER 5

MANAGEMENT OF OSTEOCHONDRAL DEFECTS: MOSAICPLASTY TECHNIQUE

LÁSZLÓ HANGODY, MD, PHD, DSC

GÁBOR K. RÁTHONYI, MD

This chapter describes the role of mosaicplasty in treating osteoarthritis (OA). While OA is a relative contraindication for mosaicplasty, indications can be widened to include salvage procedures, with the understanding that there is a higher risk of poor outcomes in this patient group.

Patients with focal chondral and osteochondral defects on the joints' loading surfaces often report pain, swelling, clicking, or instability. The defect may initiate early degenerative changes. Low-grade superficial chondral defects can be treated with nonsurgical methods such as chondroprotective medication, nonsteroidal anti-inflammatory drugs, physical therapy and balneotherapy, massage, and physiotherapy. Focal full-thickness cartilage or osteochondral defects with noninflammatory patho-origin on weight-bearing surfaces pose a great challenge for musculoskeletal specialists. Although a relatively wide range of surgical procedures has been proposed, follow-up studies report mixed results.[1-5] Several resurfacing techniques introduced in clinical practice in the last decade can be divided in two main groups. The first type of technique, so-called traditional resurfacing, results in ingrown reparative fibrocartilage. Recently introduced techniques provide hyaline or hyaline-like repair tissue that has superior biomechanical characteristics compared with reparative fibrocartilage. Several studies provide experimental data on these new resurfacing techniques, but only autologous chondrocyte transplantation and autologous osteochondral transplantation have been used extensively in clinical practice.[6-20]

We believe that the proper indication for autologous osteochondral transplantation of local full-thickness osteochondral defects depends on identification and simultaneous correction of malalignment and/or traumatic changes in affected joints. To a great extent, unfavorable outcomes may arise from improper patient selection. A better understanding of underlying pathophysiologic and biomechanical alteration will clarify the indications. Primary OA is without any identifiable causative factor, such as inflammation, trauma, metabolic changes, obesity, or altered biomechanics. By contrast, secondary osteoarthritic changes are initiated by one or a combination of the above-mentioned known factors.

The effect of structural and biomechanical changes in synovial joints has been studied extensively for many years. Correction of malalignment with osteotomy or soft-tissue release, excision or repair of meniscal tears, and ligament reconstruction has proved useful in slowing or even halting osteoarthritic changes.

PRINCIPLES OF MOSAICPLASTY

Autologous osteochondral transplantation uses multiple cylindrical grafts to fill the defect, providing a congruent, hyaline cartilage-covered surface. Some authors have reported long-term survival of the hyaline cartilage in the transplanted osteochondral block; therefore, the concept of transplanting an autologous osteochondral graft is not new.[21-24] However, clinical use of single block osteochondral transfer has been limited by congruency problems and donor site availability. According to cadaver studies and initial animal trials, multiple small-sized cylindrical graft transfer allows more tissue to be transplanted while preserving donor site integrity, and a mosaic-like implanting method permits progressive contouring of the new surface compared to a single large block graft.[25-26] Several series of animal and cadaver studies have defined the ideal donor site, graft dimension, and optimal filling rate.[27-30] According to our basic thesis, mosaic-like transplantation of multiple, small-sized cylindrical osteochondral grafts harvested from the relatively less weight-bearing periphery of the patellofemoral joint can provide a congruent resurfaced area. Survival of transplanted hyaline cartilage is very likely, and the resulting hyaline cartilage provides a more durable surface than a fibrous repair tissue. Donor tunnels are expected to fill with cancellous bone and to be covered with reparative fibrocartilage by marrow-derived cells.

Histologic Results in Experimental Studies

The mosaicplasty concept was tested in German Shepherd dogs, in horses, and in cadaver studies in preclinical phase and later experimental controls.[27-30] Macroscopic and histologic evaluations of the recipient and donor areas showed: (1) consistent survival of the transplanted hyaline cartilage; (2) formation of a composite cartilage layer from transplanted hyaline cartilage and fibrocartilage ingrown from the bony base of the defect; (3) deep matrix integration of the transplanted cartilage to the surrounding tissue at the recipient site; and (4) donor sites filled to the surface with cancellous bone and capped by fibrocartilage by 8 to 10 weeks. Fibrocartilage coverage of the donor site gave acceptable gliding surface for these less weight-bearing areas.

After successful and reproducible experimental confirmation, clinical application began on February 6, 1992. Matsusue and associates[31] and later Bobic[32] developed similar techniques for transplantation of multiple cylindrical osteochondral grafts. Clinical results reported by various authors were similar to animal results reported during the next 11 years. Since 1995, the procedure has been used with equal success at numerous clinics throughout the world, matching the favorable outcome reported by several authors' follow-up.[19,20,32-40] Recently, biomechanical testing of the press-fit technique was performed to analyze the important details of the mosaicplasty technique with further experimental studies and histologic evaluations of the recipient and donor areas.[41-45]

Surgical Technique

Mosaic-like transplantation of small-sized cylindrical osteochondral grafts (2.7, 3.5, 4.5, 6.5, and 8.5 mm in diameter) harvested by different sized cylindrical chisels from the medial or lateral margin of the medial and lateral femoral condyles superior to the sulcus terminalis and transplanted to prepared defect sites on the weight-bearing surfaces represents the main goal of the mosaicplasty technique. Notch area may serve as an additional graft harvesting site for larger defects, but special features of this area (concave chondral surface, stiffer subchondral bone) represent less favorable conditions. Implantation is performed with a step-by-step technique, which involves creation of recipient tunnels by specially sized drill bits, followed by conical shaped dilation of these holes and careful insertion of the harvested plugs. A congruent surface and 80% to 100% filling rate can be achieved with combinations of different graft sizes. Composite cartilage surface will develop by fibrocartilage grouting, stimulated by abrasion arthroplasty or sharp curettage at the base of the defect. This repair tissue cap consists of about 80% to 100% transplanted hyaline cartilage and up to 20% regenerative fibrocartilage. With the original method, donor holes are left empty and subsequently filled by cancellous bone and covered by fibrocartilage tissue in 8 to 10 weeks. Ongoing studies are evaluating different methods to fill donor tunnels and decrease postoperative bleeding.

Postoperative Rehabilitation

The postoperative rehabilitation schedule after autologous osteochondral mosaicplasty permits immediate full range of motion, but requires no weight bearing for 2 weeks and an additional 2 to 3 weeks of partial weight bearing (30 to 40 kg). The initial non–weight-bearing phase is recommended to prevent graft subsidence during osseous integration. Continuous passive motion can be used to

FIGURE 1

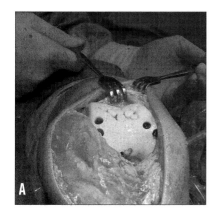 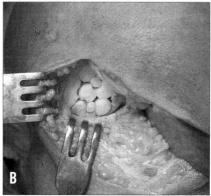 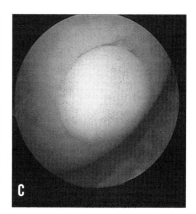

A, Open mosaicplasty on the trochlea. B, Miniarthrotomy mosaicplasty on the medial femoral condyle. C, Arthroscopic mosaicplasty on the medial femoral condyle by one 8.5-mm plug.

promote cartilage metabolism in the first 2 weeks. Further graft incorporation is secured by partial weight bearing that promotes fibrocartilage repair among the implanted cylindrical plugs. Normal daily activity can be resumed in 8 to 10 weeks. Return to a high-demand sport should be postponed for 5 to 6 months postoperatively. This protocol can be easily modified in accordance with established guidelines for concurrent anterior cruciate ligament reconstruction, high tibial osteotomy, meniscus reinsertion, and meniscus resection.

INDICATIONS FOR MOSAICPLASTY

Initial indications for autologous osteochondral mosaicplasty consist of relatively small- and medium-sized focal chondral and osteochondral defects of the weight-bearing surfaces of the femoral condyles and the patellofemoral joint (Figure 1). Later, treatment of other diarthrodial surface defects, including talar, tibial, caput and capitulum humeri, and recently, femoral head lesions, was introduced based on the successful follow-up of femoral condyle and patellofemoral mosaicplasty[30,46-49] (Figure 2). Talar mosaicplasty became popular and other authors reported promising clinical outcomes.[50-51] Matsusue and associates[52] recently reported on arthroscopic implantation on the tibial plateau. Donor site availability and other technical considerations limit the optimal extent of defect coverage to between 1 and 4 cm². Usually both of the patellofemoral peripheries allow graft harvest for 3- to 4-cm² defects. Mosaicplasty of defects up to 8 to

FIGURE 2

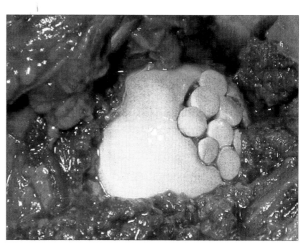

Open mosaicplasty on the femoral head.

9 cm² can be used as a salvage procedure, but extensive graft harvesting can result in higher donor site morbidity.[30] Decreased repair capacity with aging also seems to be a limiting factor. The recommended upper limit for this procedure is age 50 years based on clinical experiences with single block osteochondral transfer.[22-24]

It is important to mention that resurfacing is only one element of treatment of chondral and osteochondral defects. In every case, any accompanying joint abnormalities also must be treated because early wear of transplanted cartilage or even further degeneration is likely.

FIGURE 3

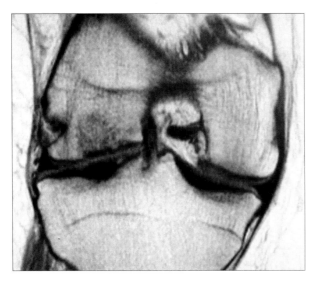

MRI scan of a 30-week-old mosaicplasty on the lateral femoral condyle in a patient who had osteochondritis dissecans of the lateral femoral condyle.

Accordingly, solutions for instabilities, malalignments, and meniscal and ligament tears must be incorporated in the surgical and postoperative rehabilitation algorithms.

CONTRAINDICATIONS FOR MOSAICPLASTY

Infection, tumors, and generalized synovial disease or rheumatoid arthritis are theoretically absolute contraindications for mosaicplasty because of the biochemical alterations that may occur in the involved joint's milieu. Mild primary OA serves as a relative contraindication since mosaicplasty is not suitable for treating generalized degenerative joint changes. In addition, OA could limit optimal quality of the donor area and have a negative effect on outcomes. However, in selected patients with mild OA, mosaicplasty can be used as a salvage procedure to avoid more invasive surgical modalities. To support this hypothesis, we analyzed our follow-up data and estimated the impact of OA on the outcome. We also analyzed follow-up data from mosaicplasty in athletic patients with borderline or salvage indications. Special demand in athletes can be measured as the ratio of return to previous sport activity. The above-mentioned subgroups represent cer-

tain extensions of normal indications.

AUTHORS' STUDY

Methods and Materials

Between February 6, 1992, and February 28, 2002, we performed 831 mosaicplasties on knees, ankles, elbows, hips, and shoulders. Of these, 597 were done on the femoral condyles, 118 on the patellofemoral joint, 76 on the talar domes, 25 on the tibial condyles, 6 on the capitulum humeri, 6 on the femoral heads, and 3 on the humeral heads. Mosaicplasty was indicated for localized grade III or IV cartilage lesion in two thirds of the patients, whereas about one third underwent surgery because of osteochondral defects.

Results of these resurfacing procedures were evaluated at regular intervals by standardized clinical scores, radiographs, and, in selected cases, by MRI (Figure 3). In certain cases, second-look arthroscopy (Figure 4), histologic evaluation of biopsy materials, and cartilage stiffness measurements were conducted. Modified Hospital for Special Surgery (HSS) and modified Cincinnati, Lysholm, and International Cartilage Repair Society (ICRS) scoring systems were used to evaluate femoral, tibial, and patellar implantations. Patients with talar lesions were evaluated using the Hannover scoring system. The Bandi scoring system was used in all cases to assess possible donor site disturbances. During the above-mentioned period, 83 second-look arthroscopies were done to check the quality of the resurfaced area and the morphologic features of the donor sites. These second-look arthroscopies were performed in 19 patients (2 months to 6 years) because of persistent or recurrent pain, swelling, or postoperative intra-articular bleeding; in 23 patients (1 to 9 years) because of a second trauma. In 41 patients, second-look arthroscopies were indicated at 4 to 7 months postoperatively to evaluate the quality of the resurfaced area and to determine the earliest date to return to the professional sports activity. In a limited series of 23 patients, cartilage stiffness measurements were performed by an arthroscopic indentometric device.

In 147 patients with existing OA, mosaicplasties were evaluated as salvage procedures and were compared with the "normal" indications. Of the 146 patients, 93 had implantations on the femoral condyles, 41 on the patella and trochlear groove, 8 on the tibial surfaces, and 5 on the talus. The main goal of this evaluation was to clarify the influence of existing degenerative joint disease on clinical outcome of the mosaicplasty procedure.

Results of autologous osteochondral mosaicplasties were also assessed in a special group of 92 high-demand professional athletes. A total of 55 men and 37 women with an average age of 26 years (range, 14 to 39 years) were included in the evaluation. Twenty-six soccer players, 16 handball players, 10 track and field athletes, 8 water polo players, 7 wrestlers, 6 gymnastic athletes, and 19 sportsmen from other fields were evaluated in this retrospective study. Evaluations were conducted for 51 medial condylar, 15 lateral condylar, 14 talar, 10 patellofemoral, 2 capitulum humeri, and 1 lateral tibial condylar defect implantations. Forty-two full-thickness osteochondral defects and 51 full-thickness chondral lesions were followed. Mild or moderate signs of OA were observed in the preoperative assessment of 43% of the patients. OA is a relative contraindication for mosaicplasty, but in this high-demand professional athlete patient group, these operations were still performed as salvage procedures. In 84 patients, the defect was smaller than 4 cm^2, but in 9 patients this limit was exceeded. Evaluations were done between 1 and 10 years postoperatively (average follow-up, 5.1 years).

Results

According to our previous evaluation[30] of the "normal" group, good to excellent results were found in 92% of patients with femoral condylar implantations, in 90% of tibial resurfacings, in 82% of patellar and/or trochlear mosaicplasties, and in 94% of talar procedures. The Bandi score showed minor donor site disturbances in 3% of patients (evaluations were done in 1- to 10-year intervals). In control patients, arthroscopy resulted in good gliding surfaces, histologically proven survival of the transplanted hyaline cartilage, and acceptable fibrocartilage covering the donor sites in 69 of the 83 patients. Slight or severe degenerative changes were seen at the recipient sites in 14 patients (four chondral lesions and 10 osteochondritis dissecans). Twenty-three patients were tested by the Artscan 1000 device (Artscan Oy, Helsinki, Finland) during control arthroscopy. During these evaluations, a computerized indentometric device performed cartilage stiffness measurements at 10 N pressure. Stiffness of the resurfaced area in most cases was similar to the surrounding, healthy hyaline cartilage.

Postoperative complications consisted of four deep infections and 36 painful hemarthroses. Arthroscopic or open débridement resolved all deep infections; 12 patients

FIGURE 4

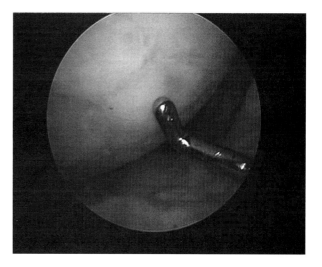

A 3-year-old mosaicplasty of the lateral femoral condyle in a patient who had a full-thickness cartilage defect.

with hemorrhaging required arthroscopic or open débridement. All other patients with hemarthroses were treated by aspiration and cryotherapy. Four patients had minor thromboembolic complications.

Patients with OA were evaluated as a subgroup and matched with the overall data to assess the effectiveness of mosaicplasty. The HSS score fell from 92 to 77 and from 90 to 69 in patients who underwent femoral and tibial condylar mosaicplasty, respectively. The Hannover score in talar mosaicplasty decreased from 94 to 88. In patients undergoing patellar and trochlear mosaicplasty, the HSS score dropped from 88 to 62. In this group of patients, donor site morbidity increased from 3% to 15% according to the Bandi score. According to our evaluation, no other complication increased with broadened indication.

Evaluation of the effectiveness of mosaicplasties in the 92 athletes was determined principally by return to sports activity and number of complications. An average of 4.9 months was spent in rehabilitation with a goal to resume sports activity at a competitive level. There were no septic or thromboembolic complications in this group. According to the return to sports activity, the following outcomes were observed: (1) 64% of the patients returned to the same level of sports activity (three participated in the Olympics in 1996 and 2000); (2) 19% returned to a lower level of sports activity, including hobby sport; and (3) 17% discontinued any kind of sports activity.

CASE STUDY

The following case study describes a typical extended indication case of mosaicplasty for Ahlback diseases in an OA patient. A 48-year-old woman was referred to our clinic with pain and swelling of the left knee. Weight-bearing radiographs showed 3° of varus malalignment and slight OA changes; MRI revealed a 6- to 8-mm deep osteochondral defect in the center of the medial femoral condyle. Arthroscopy showed a 2.5 cm² focal osteochondral defect on the medial femoral condyle and overall healthy cartilage conditions. The defect was treated with open mosaicplasty, and an open wedge high tibial osteotomy was performed to correct the malalignment. The rehabilitation schedule consisted of 3 weeks of non–weight-bearing and 3 weeks of partial weight bearing with 30 kg. Full range of motion was restored in 6 weeks, and the patient was pain free at a 3-year follow-up. The modified HSS score was 92 at both the 1-year and 3-year follow-up.

SUMMARY AND CONCLUSIONS

Mosaicplasty consisting of autologous osteochondral grafting represents an innovative and promising treatment of 1 to 4 cm² focal chondral and osteochondral articular cartilage defects. Outcomes largely depend on the adherence to proper indications, attention to technical details, and treatment of any accompanying joint abnormality.

Overall results have ranged from good to excellent, with a low complication rate in a series of more than 800 patients involving various diarthroidal joints with varying function and biomechanical loads. The procedure can be used in patients up to 50 years; however, it should be noted that patients who are younger than 50 years have faired better. Several independent evaluations reported similar results, suggesting that the technique is well standardized, and with the same indications, the results are reproducible.[31-40] Most of the evaluations are retrospective, but there are also prospective comparative follow-ups.

Appropriate treatment of the underlying causes is essential in the success of any cartilage repair technique. Success of autologous osteochondral transplantation of focal full-thickness osteochondral defects depends on identification and simultaneous correction of malalignment and/or traumatic changes in affected joints. Mosaicplasty easily allows integration of other corrective surgeries and accompanying rehabilitation protocols.

Concerns regarding donor site morbidity still remain a question. A recent biomechanical study demonstrated relatively high loading forces in the donor area, but the authors stated that until this time there is no evidence that graft harvest would result in further degenerative changes.[41] Of the entire study group, mainly transient symptoms were attributed to the donor sites. Donor site controls included patients with talar, capitellar, femoral, or humeral head lesions for whom knee surgery is performed only to procure the osteochondral plugs. These patients, with rare exception, have had no long-term knee problems. We think that full restoration of the donor site centers on the peripheral position of the donor area and the small size and proper spacing of the individual grafts. These two elements allow the joint to reconstitute structurally and to reaccept the relatively low loads in these parts of the knee.

Poor outcomes highlight the risk of broadened indication in patients with OA. However, femoral, condylar, and talar mosaicplasty can be used as a salvage procedure in these patients with only the slightest decrease in outcomes. Careful patient selection and correction of the underlying biomechanical disorders may be crucial factors to achieve a long-lasting good clinical outcome. Identification and simultaneous correction of malalignment with osteotomy or soft-tissue release, excision or repair of meniscal tears, and ligament reconstruction proved useful in slowing or even halting preexisting osteoarthritic changes.

Follow-up of high-performance competitive athletes represents a very critical form of evaluation. A relatively high proportion of these operations were performed as salvage procedures because of the presence of osteoarthritic changes (43%) and relatively extended lesions. Despite these disadvantageous conditions, this patient group still achieved an outstanding clinical outcome. Two thirds of the patients maintained their former extreme physical activity level, and only a small proportion (17%) had to discontinue sports activity. This exceptional success rate suggests that by careful and critical consideration of indications and contraindications, mosaicplasty can also be used as a salvage procedure in selected cases.

According to our encouraging results in this increasingly large series supported by similar findings from other centers, it seems that autologous osteochondral mosaicplasty may be a viable alternative treatment for localized full-thickness cartilage damage of the weight-bearing surfaces of the knee and other weight-bearing synovial joints.

In conclusion, we find that mosaicplasty has its role for treating focal osteochondral defects in patients with OA and professional athletes in selected cases as a salvage procedure.

References

1. Grana WA: Healing of articular cartilage. *Am J Knee Surg* 2000;13:29-32.
2. Buckwalter JA, Mankin HJ: Articular cartilage restoration. *Arthritis Rheum* 1998;41:1331-1342.
3. Browne JE, Branch TP: Surgical alternatives for treatment of articular cartilage lesions. *J Am Acad Orthop Surg* 2000;8:180-189.
4. Sgaglione NA, Miniaci A, Gillogly SD, Carter TR: Update on advanced surgical techniques in the treatment of traumatic focal articular lesions in the knee. *Arthroscopy* 2002;18:9-32.
5. Jackson DW, Scheer MJ, Simon TM: Cartilage substitutes: Overview of basic science and treatment options. *J Am Acad Orthop Surg* 2001;9:37-52.
6. Bruns J, Kersten P, Lierse W, Silberman M: Autologous rib perichondrial grafts in experimentally induced osteochondral lesions in the sheep-knee joint: Morphological results. *Virchows Arch A Pathol Anat Histopathol* 1992;421:1-12.
7. Coutts RD, Woo SL, Amiel D, et al: Rib perichondrial autografts in full-thickness articular cartilage defects in rabbits. *Clin Orthop* 1992;275:263-267.
8. Ritsila VA, Santavirta S, Alhopuro S, et al: Periosteal and perichondrial grafting in reconstructive surgery. *Clin Orthop* 1994;302:259
9. O'Driscoll SW, Keeley FW, Salter RB: Durability of regenerated articular cartilage produced by free autogenous periosteal grafts in major full-thickness defects in joint surfaces under the influence of continuous passive motion: A follow-up report at one year. *J Bone Joint Surg Am* 1988;70:595-606.
10. Messner K, Gillquist J: Synthetic implants for the repair of osteochondral defects of the medial femoral condyle: A biomechanical and histological evaluation in the rabbit knee. *Biomaterials* 1993;14:513-519.
11. Muckle DS, Minns RJ: Biological response to woven carbon fibre pads in the knee: A clinical and experimental study. *J Bone Joint Surg Br* 1990;72:60-62.
12. Aubin PP, Cheak HK, Davis AM, Gross AE: Long-term follow up of fresh femoral osteochondral allografts for posttraumatic knee defects. *Clin Orthop* 2001;(suppl 391): S318-S327.
13. Garrett JC: Treatment of osteochondritis dissecans of the distal femur with fresh osteochondral allografts: A preliminary report. *Arthroscopy* 1986;2:222-226.
14. Brittberg M, Lindahl A, Nilsson A, et al: Treatment of deep cartilage defects in the knee with autologous chondrocyte transplantations. *N Engl J Med* 1994;331:889-895.
15. Mandelbaum BR, Browne JE, Fu F, et al: Articular cartilage lesions of the knee. *Am J Sports Med* 1998;26:853-861.
16. Minas T: Autologous chondrocyte implantation for focal chondral defects of the knee. *Clin Orthop* 2001;(suppl 391): S349-S361.
17. Hangody L, Feczkó P, Bartha L, Bodó G, Kish G: Mosaicplasty for the treatment of articular defects of the knee and ankle. *Clin Orthop* 2001;(suppl 391):S328-S336.
18. Miller RH III: Osteochondral tissue transfers. *Am J Knee Surg* 2000;13:51-62.
19. Barber FA, Chow JCY: Arthroscopic osteochondral transplantation: Histologic results. *Arthroscopy* 2001;17:832-835.
20. Christel P, Versier G, Landreau P, Djian P: Les greffes osteo-chondrales selon la technique de la mosaicplasty. *Maitrise Orthop* 1998;76:1-13.
21. Lane JM, Brighton CT, Ottens HT, et al: Joint resurfacing in the rabbit using an autologous osteochondral graft. *J Bone Joint Surg Am* 1977;59:218-222.
22. Yamashita F, Sakakida K, Suzu F, Takai S: The transplantation of an autogenic osteochondral fragment for osteochondritis dissecans of the knee. *Clin Orthop* 1985;201:43-50.
23. Campanacci M, Cervellati C, Donati U: Autogenous patella as replacement for a resected femoral or tibial condyle: A report on 19 cases. *J Bone Joint Surg Br* 1985;67:557-563.
24. Outerbridge HK, Outerbridge AR, Outerbridge RE: The use of a lateral patellar autologous graft for the repair of a large osteochondral defect in the knee. *J Bone Joint Surg Am* 1995;77:65-72.
25. Hangody L, Kárpáti Z: New alternative in the treatment of severe, localized cartilage damages in the knee joint. *Hung J Traumat Orthop* 1994;37:237-242.
26. Hangody L, Kárpáti Z, Tóth J, et al: Autogenous osteochondral grafting in the knees of German Shepherd dogs: Radiographic and histological analysis. *Hungarian Rev Sportsmed* 1994;35:177-193.
27. Hangody L, Kish G, Kárpáti Z, et al: Autogenous osteochondral graft technique for replacing knee cartilage defects in dogs. *Orthopaedics* 1997;5:175-181.
28. Bodó G, Hangody L, Szabó Zs, Girtler D, Peham V, Schinzel M: Arthroscopic autologous osteochondral mosaicplasty for the treatment of subchondral cystic lesion in the medial femoral condyle in a horse. *Acta Vet Hung* 2000;48:343-354.
29. Bodó G, Kaposi AD, Hangody L, et al: The surgical technique and the age of the horse both influence the out-

come of mosaicplasty in a cadaver equine stifle model. *Acta Vet Hung* 2001;49:111-116.

30. Hangody L, Fules P: Autologous osteochondral mosaic-plasty for the treatment of full thickness defects of weight bearing joints: Ten years of experimental and clinical experiences. *J Bone Joint Surg Am* 2003;85(suppl 2):25-32.

31. Matsusue Y, Yamamuro T, Hama H: Arthroscopic multiple osteochondral transplantation to the chondral defect in the knee associated with anterior cruciate ligament disruption-case report. *Arthroscopy* 1993;9:318.

32. Bobic V: Arthroscopic osteochondral autogenous graft transplantation in anterior cruciate reconstruction: A preliminary report. *Knee Surg Sports Traumatol Arthrosc* 1996;3:262.

33. Imhoff AB, Ottl GM, Burkart A, Traub S: Autologous osteochondral transplantation on various joints. *Orthopade* 1999;28:33-44.

34. Berlet GC, Mascia A, Miniaci A: Treatment of unstable osteochondritis dissecans lesions of the knee using autogenous osteochondral grafts (mosaicplasty). *Arthroscopy* 1999;15:312-316.

35. Solheim E: Mosaikkplastikk ved leddbruskskader i kne. *Tidsskr Nor Laegeforen* 1999;27:4022-4025.

36. Marcacci M, Kon E, Zaffagnini S, Visani A: Use of autologous grafts for reconstruction of osteochondral defects of the knee. *Orthopedics* 1999;22:595-600.

37. Traub S, Imhoff AB, Öttl G: Die Technik der osteochondralen autologen Knorpeltransplantation (OATS) zum Ersatz chondraler oder osteochondraler Defekte. *Osteologie* 2000;9:46-55.

38. Maynou C, Mestdagh H, Beltrand E, et al: Resultats a long term de l'autogreffe osteo-cartilagineuse de voisinage dans les destructions cartilagineuses etendues du genou. A propos de 5 cas. *Acta Orthop Belg* 1998;64:193-2000.

39. Ripoli PL, de Prado M, Ruiz D, Salmeron J: Transplantes osteocondrales en mosaico: estudio de los resultados mediante RMN y segunda artroscopia. *Cuadernos Artroscopia* 2000;6:11-16.

40. Attmanspacher W, Dittrich V, Stedtfeld HW: Experiences with arthroscopic therapy of chondral and osteochondral defects of the knee joint with OATS (Osteochondral Autograft Transfer System). *Zentralbl Chir* 2000;125: 494-499.

41. Simonian PT, Sussmann PS, Wiczkiewicz TL, et al: Contact pressures at osteochondral donor sites in the knee. *Am J Sports Med* 1998;26:491-494.

42. Duchow J, Hess T, Kohn D: Primary stability of press-fit-implanted osteochondral grafts. *Am J Sports Med* 2000;28:24-27.

43. Hurtig M, Pearce S, Warren M, Kalra M, Miniaci A: Arthroscopic mosaic arthroplasty in the equine third carpal bone. *Vet Surg* 2001;30:228-239.

44. Makino T, Fujioka H, Kurosaka M, et al: Histologic analysis of the implanted cartilage in an exact-fit osteochondral transplantation model. *Arthroscopy* 2001;17:747-751.

45. Ahmad CS, Guiney WB, Drinkwater CJ: Evaluation of donor site intrinsic healing response in autologous osteochondral grafting of the knee. *Arthroscopy* 2002;18:95-98.

46. Hangody L, Kish G, Kárpáti Z, et al: Mosaicplasty for the treatment of articular cartilage defects: Application in clinical practice. *Orthopaedics* 1998;21:751-758.

47. Hangody L, Kish G, Kárpáti Z, Szerb I, Eberhardt R: Treatment of osteochondritis dissecans of the talus: Use of the mosaicplasty technique. A preliminary report. *Foot Ankle Int* 1997;18:628-634.

48. Hangody L, Kish G, Kárpáti Z, et al: Two to seven year results of autologous osteochondral mosaicplasty on the talus. *Foot Ankle Int* 2001;22:552-558.

49. Hidas P, Hangody L, Csépai D, Pavlik A, Pantó T: Mosaikplastik: Eine neue Alternative in der Behandlung der Osteochondritis dissecans des Capitulum humeri. *Arthroskopie* 2002;15:59-63.

50. Assenmacher JA, Kelikian AS, Gottlob C, Kodros S: Arthroscopically assisted autologous osteochondral transplantation for osteochondral lesions of the talar dome: An MRI and clinical follow-up study. *Foot Ankle Int* 2001;22:544-551.

51. Kish G: Mosaicplasty for osteochondral lesions of the talus, in Kitaoka HB (ed): *Master Techniques in Orthopaedic Surgery: The Foot and Ankle*. Philadelphia, PA, Lippincott-Williams-Wilkins, 2002, pp 643-664.

52. Matsusue Y, Kotake T, Nakagawa Y, Nakamura T: Arthroscopic osteochondral autograft transplantation for chondral lesion of the tibial plateau of the knee. *Arthroscopy* 2001;17:653-659.

CHAPTER 6

SECOND-GENERATION ACI TECHNIQUE

MAURILIO MARCACCI, MD
STEFANO ZAFFAGNINI, MD
ELIZAVETA KON, MD
ALBERTO VASCELLARI, MD

Finding an efficient means for treating full-thickness lesions of the articular surface in the knee remains a challenge for the orthopaedic surgeon. Identifying the exact lesion in need of repair remains a challenge as well. The marked increase in both sports participation and general physical activity in all age groups has also increased the incidence of these lesions and the recovery expectations of patients. However, articular cartilage lesions are difficult to treat given their distinctive structure, the function of hyaline cartilage, and ultimately the difficulty in identifying which lesions will be symptomatic and eventually cause degenerative joint changes. In their review of 31,516 knee arthroscopies, Curl and associates[1] found a 63% incidence of chondral lesions in which 20% were grade IV lesions but 35% had no accompanying meniscal or ligamentous lesions. Their results emphasize the difficulty in identifying which tissue injury is responsible for which symptoms and to what extent. Messner and Maletius[2] reported good to excellent clinical results without treatment in 22 of 28 patients with isolated, asymptomatic chondral lesions; however, most of their patients had abnormal radiographic changes on presentation and progressive degeneration of the knee joint. Thus, it would appear that Hunter's assertion in 1743 that cartilage "once destroyed is not repaired" remains essentially true, and many current authors agree.[3-5]

APPROACHES TO CARTILAGE REPAIR

Isolated injuries to the cartilage of the knee increase the risk for more extensive joint damage because the intrinsic capacity of cartilage to repair itself is limited, given its isolation from systemic regulation and its lack of vessels and nerve supply.[3,6-8] None of the inflammatory processes is available for cartilage repair, and chondrocytes, unlike most tissue, cannot migrate to the site of injury from an intact, healthy site.[3,7] These obstacles to self-repair stem from the unique architecture and ultrastructure of articular cartilage in which chondrocytes are sparsely distributed within the surrounding matrix, thereby maintaining minimal cell-to-cell contact. The interactions among the cells, collagen framework, aggrecan, and fluid constitute the complex biomechanical feature of hyaline cartilage, making it difficult to replace or reproduce.

Treatment options have been directed at the recruitment of bone marrow cells to obtain potential cartilage precursors. Continuous passive motion or arthroscopic lavage has been shown to be ineffective.[6] A variety of marrow stimulation techniques have been developed to allow stem cell migration from the marrow cavity to the fibrin

> One or more of the authors or the departments with which they are affiliated have received something of value from a commercial or other party related directly or indirectly to the subject of this chapter.

clot of the defect.[9] However, treatment options such as abrasion, drilling, and microfracture technique produce a predominantly fibrous repair tissue, with mostly type I collagen fibrocytes and an unorganized matrix.[9,10] Moreover, the fibrocartilage-like repair tissue lacks the biomechanical and viscoelastic characteristics of normal hyaline cartilage.[3,9] Recently Steadman and associates[11] reported highly satisfactory results at 11 years follow-up with microfracture technique; however, their results might suggest that their patients adjusted their activity level to that of their knee function. The authors also stressed the importance of a meticulous postoperative program that included continuous passive motion and 8 weeks of restricted weight bearing. Microfracture technique is simple, but the response of the repaired tissue can be unpredictable and variable; in addition, it remains unclear which stresses are optimal for cartilage regeneration. Nehrer and associates[12] frequently found fibrous, soft, spongiform tissue combined with central degeneration in the defect. They reported clinical failure several months after treatment (mean, 21 months). These techniques for repairing cartilage defects have been partially successful in reducing pain and increasing mobility. However, the failure rate is quite high, and no well-established solution to this problem has been presented.

Osteochondral autograft transfer, as proposed by Hangody and associates,[13] can be considered a secondary procedure for treating symptomatic unipolar grade IV distal femoral condyle lesions between 1 and 2.5 cm in diameter. This technique is technically demanding, and the location of the donor site and the size of the harvested grafts play a key role in its success. Achieving complete coverage of the defect, mechanical stability of the plugs, and restoration to a level congruent with that of healthy cartilage are critical factors and difficult to achieve. Because the availability of this type of autologous graft is limited, this procedure is not commonly used.

AUTOLOGOUS CHONDROCYTE IMPLANTATION

History

Autologous chondrocyte implantation (ACI) was first used in the early 1980s. Several studies have shown that chondrocyte reproduction can be stimulated in vitro,[14] and animal studies have demonstrated the production of hyaline-like repair tissue when cultured chondrocytes were implanted.[10] The clinical use of ACI for treating chronic symptoms of cartilage lesions was pioneered in Sweden in 1987.[9]

The first clinical report in 1994[15] reported highly satisfactory results, with biopsy samples showing hyaline-like cartilage. Since its introduction in Sweden, ACI has gained increasing acceptance as a technique to restore articular cartilage. Several researchers have reported encouraging early clinical results, especially with lesions in the femoral condyle.[10] In this technique, a periosteal flap was used to create a vacuum chamber around the defect into which the cultured condrocytes were injected. A wide exposure is needed to create the flap; closing this exposure requires numerous stitches over the defect area.

Peterson and associates[10] recently described the durability of early results obtained with ACI. After 2 years, 50 of 61 patients reported good to excellent results. At 5- to 11-year follow-up, 51 of 61 patients still reported satisfactory results. Biomechanical evaluation of the grafted area (by means of indentation probe) demonstrated a stiffness measurement of 90% or more of the value found in the control group. These authors reported that 84% to 91% of patients achieved good to excellent results and returned to their active lifestyles. Thus, we agree with Sgaglione and associates[6] that ACI is a safe, effective, and reproducible treatment that should be considered a viable option for young patients with cartilage lesions greater than 2 cm[2]. ACI is particularly appropriate for young patients who want to resume an active lifestyle and for which restoration of so-called "normal" cartilage is a goal.

Intraoperative Problems

A variety of intraoperative challenges have prompted researchers to strive to improve the efficacy and reduce the morbidity associated with ACI. First, the liquid cell suspension is difficult to handle intraoperatively and needs to be covered by a periosteal flap, which can be detrimental to the procedure for several reasons. Stitching the periosteal flap is long, tedious, and often very difficult. A large joint exposure is also usually necessary, depending on the location of the defect. These factors increase morbidity, specifically the risk of joint stiffness and arthrofibrosis.

Recently, Micheli and associates[16] and others[17-19] reported a revision rate of up to 42% in patients with joint stiffness following ACI. Another common reason for revision surgery is the hypertrophic changes that occur as a result of the intrinsic growth capacity of the cambium layer of the periosteal flap, with impingement syndrome as an eventual development.[17-19]

Another critical point is to ensure a vacuum seal of the camera to avoid leakage from the defect of the implanted chondrocyte during the early mobilization phase or after resumption of load bearing. Excessive bleeding inside the defect causes the implanted chondrocyte to burst due to excessive pressure within the cavity, ultimately causing the procedure to fail.

Along with problems associated with the surgical procedure, there are technical problems with the culture and transplantation procedures. Maintaining the chondrocytic phenotype during a prolonged monolayer culture is critical. Chondrocytes tend to lose their ability to form matrix and produce mainly collagen type I.[3] It is still unclear whether transplanted cells reexpress their phenotype after transplantation in suspension. Another concern is whether chondrocytes are distributed in the three-dimensional space of the defect.[3]

Three-dimensional Cartilage Regeneration

After considering all of the previously described factors, we have used a new tissue engineering technology to create cartilage-like tissue in a three-dimensional culture system in an attempt to address all the concerns related to the cell culture and the surgical technique. In vitro three-dimensional cartilage regeneration is performed with chondrocytes seeded onto a bioresorbable polymeric scaffold. Hyaluronan (hyaluronic acid) appears to be an ideal candidate for tissue engineering strategies because it can function as both a structural and informational molecule. Hyaluronan is a glycosaminoglycan ubiquitously distributed in the extracellular space, especially in the extracellular matrix.[20] HYAFF is a class of hyaluronan derivates obtained by esterifying the glucuronic acid group with different types of alcohols.[21] HYAFF-11–based scaffolds can be used in skeletal tissue engineering as both a tissue guiding device and a delivery vehicle.[22]

Testing Tissue Engineering Strategies

To assess the ability to enhance natural healing, HYAFF-11 was tested in an in vivo articular defect model. Osteochondral defects were created in the femoral condyle of young adult rabbits; defects were left untreated or filled with HYAFF-11–based scaffolds. Treated defects scored significantly higher than untreated defects by exhibiting good bone filling and hyaline cartilage at the surface. Moreover, independently of the form used, hyaluronan-

based scaffolds provided consistent neo- and host-tissue integration.[23] Additional studies have been undertaken to explore the possibility to engineer tissue-combining hyaluronan-based scaffolds with cells. To improve tissue reconstruction, the use of mesenchymal progenitor cells (MPCs) has been proposed.[24] Hyaluronan-based scaffolds demonstrated MPC attachment, proliferation, and differentiation along osteochondral lineage.[25,26]

The maintenance of mature phenotypes is favored by the use of a three-dimensional scaffold. HYAFF-11 non-woven matrix has been described extensively in a series of in vitro and in vivo studies where it has been shown to effectively support growth of chondrocytes and to favor the expression of typical chondrocyte markers.[27] HYAFF-11 nonwoven mesh was shown to support the growth of human chondrocytes and to maintain their original phenotype in vitro.[28] More recently, tissue-specific gene expression was shown in chondrocytes grown on HYAFF-11–based scaffolds.[29] These findings further confirmed that a three-dimensional HYAFF-11 culture system is an effective chondrocyte delivery system for the treatment of articular cartilage defects.

To verify the potential use of HYAFF-11–based engineered cartilage in a clinical setting, a rabbit model of surgically created full-thickness defects of the medial femoral condyle was used.[30] Histologic samples from in and around the defect sites were examined and scored 1, 3, and 6 months after surgery. Statistically significant differences in the quality of the regenerated tissue were found between the grafts performed with biomaterial-carrying chondrocyte cells compared with grafts consisting of biomaterial alone or controls, thus demonstrating the efficacy of HYAFF-11–based scaffold for ACI.

Incorporating HYAFF into ACI

With this scientific and promising background, we have started using HYAFF in ACI to treat symptomatic cartilage lesions. At first we used the scaffold via a mini-open surgical approach, depending on the location of the defect, and applied the patch with fibrin glue without providing periosteal coverage. Over time, we learned that if the patch is correctly positioned inside the prepared defect, a tensioactive pressure permits natural fixation without use of any other device. A histologic sample harvested 4 months after an open implant confirmed that the scaffold is resorbable and remains in the defect (Figure 1). The ease with which this patch can be handled (without need for liquid solution or a periosteal flap) has permitted us to

FIGURE 1

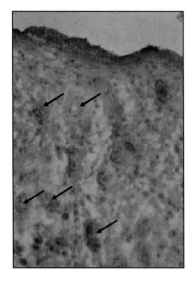

Histologic sample 4 months after Hyalograft C implant, stained for collagen type II. The giant cell agglomeration suggests reabsorption of residual hyaluronic acid fibers (arrows). (Courtesy of Dr. D. Brochetta (Monza) Hystological evaluation: Prof. G. Abbatangelo, Istituto di Anatomia, Università di Padova.)

FIGURE 2

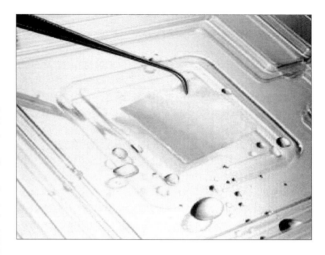

Hyalograft C implant ready for surgical application.

quickly develop an arthroscopic implant procedure to simplify and reduce morbidity associated with this two-stage procedure. Depending on the location of the defect, either a mini-open or arthroscopic approach can be used.

Mini-open Surgical Technique

The mini-open surgical technique for ACI consists of two steps: (1) biopsy of healthy cartilage to obtain autologous chondrocyte cell culture, followed by (2) implantation of the graft. The biopsy is usually performed arthroscopically when the chondral lesion is identified and ACI has been selected as treatment. Small specimens (100 mg) of healthy cartilage are harvested from the superior aspect of the intercondylar notch for cell culture. The graft is implanted after the cell culture is obtained, usually after at least 4 to 6 weeks, to ensure a well-matured graft (Figure 2).

The open surgical technique includes a mini-arthrotomy, preparation of the defect site, sizing of the graft, and implantation of the cultured graft. The dimensions of the exposure depend on the size and the location of the defect; we prefer a medial parapatellar incision for defects of the medial compartment and patellar chondral lesions and a lateral parapatellar incision for lateral sites. Visualization of the defect is necessary to prepare the site of the defect. The subchondral bone must be exposed, removing all damaged cartilage without damaging the subchondral layer. It is imperative to leave a sharp rim of healthy cartilage around the defect area. The subchondral

bone has to be exposed to avoid any lesion and to maintain hemostasis in the defect area. The defect is then measured, and a Hyalograft C (HYAFF cell) graft (FAB, Padua, Italy) is prepared matching the defect dimensions. The graft must be completely inside the margins of the defect to guarantee graft stability and to avoid any possible mobilization. The graft is then placed in the defect and its stability evaluated after flexion and extension of the knee. The wound and skin are then closed in a standard manner.

Arthroscopic Surgical Technique

The arthroscopic surgical technique for ACI also consists of two steps: (1) arthroscopic biopsy of healthy cartilage for cell culture, followed by (2) preparing the site and implanting the graft. This first step is the same as that used for open surgical technique. Note that at this time, associated procedures such as anterior cruciate ligament (ACL) reconstruction or meniscal surgeries are usually performed. The arthroscopic implant procedure was developed for use on medial or lateral condyle lesions. Over time and with experience we can now address almost every site of a grade IV defect that has a wide extension.

Under arthroscopic control, the lesion is visualized (Figure 3) and then débrided and cleaned with a motorized shaver, removing all fibrous tissue from its surface. The defect is then mapped and sized using a device with a variably sized diameter (6.5 to 8.5 mm) and sharp edges; the device should completely cover the defect (Figure 4). A cannula is then inserted into the anteromedial portal,

FIGURE 3

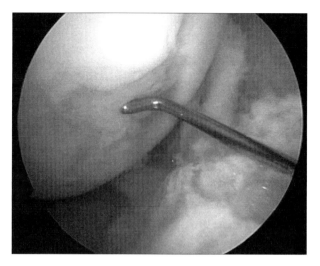

Visualization of the chondral lesion in the medial femoral condyle.

FIGURE 4

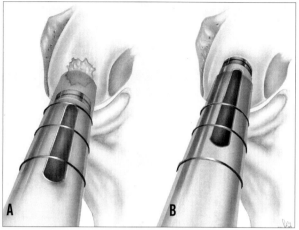

The lesion is **(A)** sized and mapped with the sharp edge of the device to ensure complete coverage **(B)**.

FIGURE 5

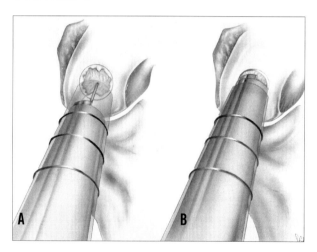

A specially designed low-profile, slow-speed drill is positioned over the defect **(A)**, avoiding the lesion of the subchondral bone **(B)**.

and a specially designed cannulated low-profile drill (6.5 to 8.5 mm) is properly positioned (Figure 5).

The drill is maintained in the selected position by a Kirschner (K-wire) guide wire (0.9-mm diameter) fixed in the bone. This drill was developed specifically with a safety stop at 2 mm to avoid damaging the subchondral bone plate because the bone plate should be left intact during débridement.[10] The K-wire passes through the subchondral plate, but the number of stem cells that escape from this small hole is not significant enough to modify the action of the cultured chondrocyte. The low-speed drilling of the cartilage surface creates a circular area with regular margins in preparation for the graft (Figure 6). The procedure is repeated to prepare the entire surface of the defect.

From the same portal, it is usually possible to correctly prepare an area that is wide enough for the graft by flexing the knee and changing the orientation of the cannula. After drilling, joint lavage is performed with a motorized shaver. The inflow is then closed and the area suctioned with the cannula to create a dry joint surface.

The hyaluronic acid patch containing the autologous chondrocyte culture is then harvested with the sharp edge of the device (Figure 7). The stamp obtained remains automatically in the sheath of the device and then is transported through a cannula and positioned in the prepared area. The delivery tamp is pushed to plug the stamp precisely in the defect (Figure 8). The procedure is repeated

until the entire defect is completely filled (Figure 9).

As much of the prepared area as possible should be covered with implanted stamps without covering the margin of the defect. In this manner, the stamps do not move from the defect. This technique has been tested after repeated cycles of joint motion (with and without the use of a tourniquet) performed in open techniques previously executed using the same device.

FIGURE 6

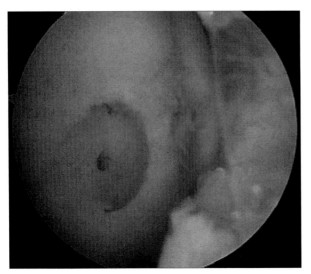

The prepared surface of the chondral lesion after drilling.

FIGURE 7

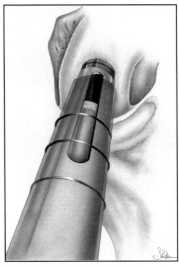

The tamp is pushed in the device to plug the stamp precisely into the defect.

The stability of implanted stamps should be evaluated with a blunt probe under arthroscopic control. Once the tourniquet is released, graft swelling and stability can be reevaluated (Figure 10). If swelling increases the size of the graft so much that the margins of the defect are covered, it is possible to insert a 6.5-mm diameter patch into an 8-mm diameter area to fill the defect without covering the margins. With the arthroscope still in place, cyclic bending of the knee should ensue so that eventual movement of the grafts from the prepared defect can be checked. We have never observed mobilization of the implanted patch.

Rehabilitation Protocol

Patients are discharged 1 day after the arthroscopic procedure and 2 days after the open procedure. From the second postoperative day through the first 2 weeks, continuous self-assisted passive motion from 0° to 90° is started to promote joint nutrition and prevent adhesions. Stretching exercises and quadriceps contractions are allowed as tolerated. Foot-touch weight bearing is permitted, whereas complete weight bearing is not allowed for the first 4 weeks.

After the first 4 to 5 weeks, weight bearing can be increased, beginning in the swimming pool, to restore normal gait. Strengthening exercises are allowed from week 7. Increased strength and functional exercises are then gradually allowed. Return to sports involving cutting and contact sports should not be attempted for at least 12 months.

CASE STUDY: RIZZOLI ORTHOPAEDIC INSTITUTE

Patient Selection

The Hyalograft C implant has been used at our institution since September 1999 in 105 patients (70 males, 35 females). Of these, 62 were treated arthroscopically (beginning in November 2000) and 43 were treated with an open surgical technique. The approval of the Ethical Committee of the Rizzoli Orthopaedic Institute was obtained for the clinical study, and an informed consent was required of all patients. All patients were evaluated prospectively according to the International Cartilage Repair Society (ICRS) score criteria—preoperatively and at 6, 12, 24, and 36 months. We obtained CT or MRI scans in all patients at 6, 12, 24, and 36 months' follow-up.

In April 2003, 58 patients (44 male, 14 female) were evaluated after at least 1 year, 32 patients at 2 years' follow-up, and 5 patients at 3 years' follow-up. Of these patients evaluated at 12 months, 52 had isolated chondral lesions, 30 had medial condyle lesions, 12 had patellar lesions, 9 had lateral condyle lesions, and 1 patient had an ankle lesion. Six patients had multiple knee lesions: two

FIGURE 8

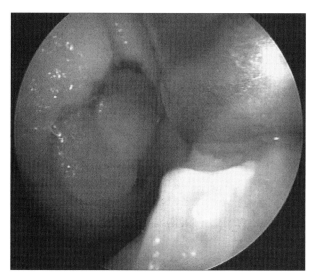

Complete coverage of the defect by two implanted patches after irrigation of the joint has been stopped.

FIGURE 9

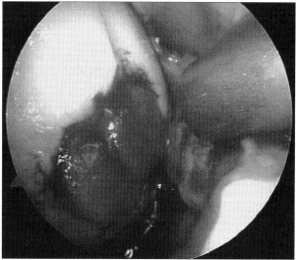

After tourniquet release and joint mobilization, the stability of the implanted patches should be evaluated.

had medial and lateral femoral condyle lesions; two had compartment "kissing" lesions (one medial, one lateral); one had a lateral compartment lesion associated with a medial condyle defect; and one had medial condyle and trochlear defects. All defects were Outerbridge grade III to IV (mean size, 3.1 cm^2 [2 to 5.7 cm^2]). Mean patient age at the time of surgery was 27.5 years (range, 15 to 43 years). The etiology was degenerative in 33 patients; traumatic in 19 patients (9 were acute and 10 were chronic), and a result of osteochondritis dissecans in 5 patients.

Of the 58 patients evaluated at the 12-month follow-up, 29 underwent the arthroscopic technique and the other 29 underwent an open technique. All patellar and tibial plateau lesions were treated with open surgery. In 26 patients, associated procedures were performed during cartilage harvesting: 13 ACL reconstructions; 11 medial and 5 lateral meniscectomies; 4 patellar realignments; 2 high tibial osteotomies; 2 procedures to remove loose bodies; 2 meniscal suture procedures; 1 collagen meniscus implant; and 1 autologous bone grafting. Previous surgery in this group of patients included 12 cartilage reparative operations, such as shaving and débridement of chondral lesions, 10 meniscectomies, 8 ACL reconstructions, 4 mosaicplasties, 1 LCP reconstruction, and 1 osteosynthesis for patellar fracture.

Follow-up Evaluations

Patients were asked to evaluate their symptoms and physical function using the International Knee Document Committee's (IKDC) Subjective Knee Evaluation Form. According to this questionnaire, a high score represents higher levels of function and lower levels of symptoms. A score of 100 means no limitations on activities of daily living or sports and the absence of symptoms. A total of 93% of the 12-month follow-up group (n = 58) reported improved knee function and symptoms; only four patients (7%) reported no change in condition. The mean IKDC Subjective Knee Evaluation Form score was 35.5 (SD = 9.8) preoperatively and 76.4 (SD = 16.5) at the 12-month follow-up.

Patients were also asked to evaluate quality of life using the EuroQol (EQ-5D) questionnaire.[31] This instrument is a recognized assessment of health-related quality of life based on self-care, mobility, usual activities, pain/discomfort, and anxiety/depression dimensions. It also includes a 0 to 100 Visual Analogue Scale (EQ-VAS) for a self-rating of global health state in which 100 represents the best imaginable health state. A total of 90% of the patients reported improved quality of life as assessed by the EQ-VAS, and 10% reported no change. EQ-VAS scores increased from 71.5 (SD = 16.8) to 91.5 (SD = 5.3) at the

FIGURE 10

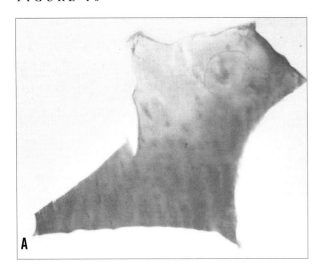 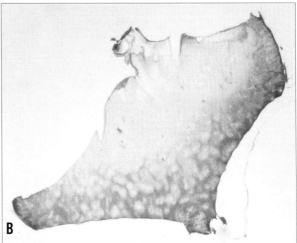

Histologic evaluation of regenerated tissue at the 12-month follow-up (Courtesy of Prof. A. Hollander, University of Bristol, UK). **A,** Biopsy specimen with safranin O staining shows intense glycosaminoglycan deposition, starting from the deeper area of the implant. In this area, chondrocyte-like cells are surrounded by lacunae, whereas on the external layers of the tissue, cells are still undergoing differentiation and cartilage matrix is still remodeling (original magnification x25). **B,** Immunolocalization of collagen type II (HRP detection). Intense staining was found starting from the inner part of the biopsy specimen. Note that the core contains moderate to few numbers of cells, whereas the surface of the specimen has a higher concentration of cells (original magnification x25).

12-month follow-up. Most of the improvements were in mobility (65%), usual activities (43%), and reduced pain/discomfort (90%); no patients reported that their condition deteriorated.

Knee function tests were also performed using the IKDC Knee Examination Form. The lowest ratings in effusion, passive motion deficit, and ligament examination were used to assign a final functional grade (normal, nearly normal, abnormal, or severely abnormal). No complications related to the implant or serious adverse events were observed during the treatment and follow-up period.

Data from the ICRS form showed that, overall, 85.5% of patents had normal (41.4%) or nearly normal (43.1%) function. Only one patient had the worst score (abnormal). Overall, at the 12-month follow-up, patients who had the arthroscopic technique faired better than those who had open surgery. Patients treated arthroscopically had good to excellent clinical results (89.6%) compared with those who had an open technique (79.3%). This difference could be partially related to the slightly different size of the defect and by the higher number of patellar lesions in the open group. Good to excellent results also were seen in patients with medial condyle lesions (83.3%), lateral condyle lesions (88.9%), and patellar lesions (75%). All six patients with multiple chondral lesions had good or excellent results. Thirty-two patients were examined at 12 and 24 months; of these, three improved and two became worse in the time between the 12- and 24-month follow-up.

A second-look arthroscopy was performed as part of follow-up evaluation in 11 patients at the 12-month follow-up and in 1 patient at 24-month follow-up. A visual check and probing for consistency of the implant showed complete healing of the defect and excellent quality of regenerated cartilage on macroscopic examination. A biopsy specimen of implanted cartilage was obtained in 25 patients (the 12 described above plus 13 from other centers), and histologic evaluation by an independent examiner showed hyaline-like tissue with good integration within the host tissue in 85% of the biopsy specimens[32] (Figure 11).

Conclusions

The results of our series are comparable to those obtained with the original ACI techniques.[9] However, with our technique, morbidity, recovery time, and the duration of the rehabilitation protocol are reduced and more acceptable to patients. In our series of patients who had either open surgery or an arthroscopic procedure, only one patient required revision for clinical symptoms. Our technique provides good clinical and histologic results, reduces morbidity, and improves the reliability of the procedure. Certainly further improvements are needed, specifically the availability of higher-quality, cartilage-like tissue with better durability. Improvements to tissue could be achieved by using chemical factors or genetic induction. Longer follow-up data on patients are also needed to demonstrate the real advantages of this technique compared to ACI.

REFERENCES

1. Curl WW, Krome J, Gordon ES, Rushing J, Smith BP, Poehling GG: Cartilage injuries: A review of 31,516 knee arthroscopies. *Arthroscopy* 1997;13:456-460.

2. Messner K, Maletius W. The long-term prognosis for severe damage to weight-bearing cartilage in the knee: A 14-year clinical and radiographic follow-up in 28 young athletes. *Acta Orthop Scand* 1996;67:165-168.

3. Ochi M, Uchio Y, Kawasaki K, Wakitani S, Iwasa J: Transplantation of cartilage-like tissue made by tissue engineering in the treatment of cartilage defects of the knee. *J Bone Joint Surg Br* 2002;84:571-578.

4. Minas T: Autologous chondrocyte implantation for focal chondral defects of the knee. *Clin Orthop* 2001; (suppl 391): S349-S361.

5. Browne JE, Branch TP: Surgical alternatives for treatment of articular cartilage lesions. *J Am Acad Orthop Surg* 2000;8:180-189.

6. Sgaglione NA, Miniaci A, Gillogly SD, Carter TR: Update on advanced surgical techniques in the treatment of traumatic focal articular cartilage lesions in the knee. *Arthroscopy* 2002;18(suppl 1):9-32.

7. Buckwalter JA, Mankin HJ: Articular cartilage. *J Bone Joint Surg Am* 1997;79:600-611.

8. Buckwalter JA, Mankin HJ: Articular cartilage: Part II. Degeneration and osteoarthrosis, repair, regeneration, and tranplantation. *J Bone Joint Surg Am* 1997;79:612-632.

9. Peterson L, Minas T, Brittberg M, Nilsson A, Sjogren-Jansson E, Lindahl A: Two- to 9-year outcome after autologous chondrocyte transplantation of the knee. *Clin Orthop* 2000;374:212-234.

10. Peterson L, Brittberg M, Kiviranta I, Akerlund EL, Lindahl A: Autologous chondrocyte transplantation: Biomechanics and long-term durability. *Am J Sports Med* 2002;30:2-12.

11. Steadman JR, Briggs KK, Rodrigo JJ, Kocher MS, Gill TJ, Rodkey WG: Outcomes of microfracture for traumatic chondral defects of the knee: Average 11-year follow-up. *Arthroscopy* 2003;19:477-484.

12. Nehrer S, Spector M, Minas T: Histologic analysis of tissue after failed cartilage repair procedures. *Clin Orthop* 1999;365:149-162.

13. Hangody L, Kish G, Karpati Z, Udvarhelyi I, Szigeti I, Bely M: Mosaicplasty for the treatment of articular cartilage defects: Application in clinical practice. *Orthopedics* 1998;21:751-756.

14. Brittberg M, Tallheden T, Sjogren-Jansson B, Lindahl A, Peterson L: Autologous chondrocytes used for articular cartilage repair: An update. *Clin Orthop* 2001;(Suppl 391): S337-S348.

15. Brittberg M, Lindahl A, Nilsson A, Ohlsson C, Isaksson O, Peterson L: Treatment of deep cartilage defects in the knee with autologous chondrocyte transplantation. *N Engl J Med* 1994;331:889-895.

16. Micheli LJ, Browne JE, Erggelet C, et al: Autologous chondrocyte implantation of the knee: Multicenter experience and minimum 3-year follow-up. *Clin J Sport Med* 2001;11:223-228.

17. Anderson AF, Fu FH, Mandelbaum BR, et al: A controlled study of autologous chondrocyte implantation versus microfracture for articular cartilage lesions of the femur. *70th Annual Meeting Proceedings.* Rosemont, IL, American Academy of Orthopaedic Surgeons, 2003, p 554.

18. Moseley JB, Micheli LJ, Erggelet C, et al: 6-year patient outcomes with autologous chondrocyte implantation. *70th Annual Meeting Proceedings.* Rosemont, IL, American Academy of Orthopaedic Surgeons, 2003, p 555.

19. Cole BJ, Nho SJ, Beddow SA, Sasso LM, DiMasi M, Hayden JK: Prospective evaluation of autologous chondrocyte implantation. *70th Annual Meeting Proceedings.* Rosemont, IL, American Academy of Orthopaedic Surgeons, 2003, p 556.

20. Abatangelo G, O'Regan M: Hyaluronan: Biological role and function in articular joints. *Eur J Rheumatol Infla* 1995;15:9-16.

21. Campoccia D, Doherty P, Radice M, Brun P, Abatangelo G, Williams DF: Semi synthetic resorbable materials from hyaluronan esterification. *Biomaterials* 1998,19:2101-2127.

22. New frontiers in medical sciences: Redefining hyaluronan. Abatangelo G, Weigel PH (eds): Proceedings of the Symposium held in Padua, Italy, June 17-19, 1999. Elsevier, 2000.

23. Solchaga LA, Yoo JU, Lundberg M, et al: Hyaluronan-based polymers in the treatment of osteochondral defects. *J Orthop Res* 2000;18:773-780.

24. Caplan AI, Bruder SP: Mesenchymal stem cells: Building blocks for molecular medicine in the 21st century. *Trends Molec Med* 2001;7:259-264.

25. Solchaga LA, Dennis JE, Goldberg VM, Caplan AI: Hyaluronic acid-based polymers as cell carriers for tissue-engineered repair of bone and cartilage. *J Orthop Res* 1999;17:205-213.

26. Radice M, Brun P, Cortivo R, Scapinelli R, Battaliard C, Abatangelo G: Hyaluronan-based biopolymers as delivery vehicles for bone-marrow-derived mesenchymal progenitors. *J Biomed Mater Res* 2000;50:101-109.

27. Brun P, Abatangelo G, Radice M, et al: Chondrocyte aggregation and reorganization into three-dimensional scaffolds. *J Biomed Mater Res* 1999;46:337-346.

28. Grigolo B, Lisignoli G, Piacentini A, et al: Evidence for redifferentiation of human chondrocytes grown on a hyaluronan-based biomaterial (HYAFF®11). *Biomaterials* 2002;23:1187-1195.

29. Girotto D, Urbani S, Brun P, Renier D, Barbucci R, Abatangelo G: Tissue-specific gene expression in chondrocytes grown on three-dimensional hyaluronic acid scaffolds. *Biomaterials* 2003;24:3265-3275.

30. Grigolo B, Roseti L, Fiorini M, et al: Transplantation of chondrocytes seeded on a hyaluronan derivative (HYAFF®11) into cartilage defects in rabbits. *Biomaterials* 2001;22:2417-2424.

31. Rabin R, de Charro F. EQ-5D: A measure of health status from the EuroQol Group. *Ann Med* 2001;33:337-343.

32. Marcacci M, Kon E, Zaffagnini S, Abatangelo G: Autologous chondrocyte transplantation on 3-dimensional hyaluronic acid support (Hyalograft C): Histologic evaluation at 1 year follow-up. Paper presented at AOSSM Specialty Day, February 8, 2003, New Orleans, LA.

CHAPTER 7

UNICONDYLAR KNEE ARTHROPLASTY: BENEFITS AND PITFALLS

PHILIPPE CARTIER, MD

ARTHROPLASTY STUDY

Between 1974 and 2003, my colleagues and I implanted 1,941 unicompartmental prostheses, starting with Marmor prostheses (Richards, Smith & Nephew, Memphis, TN), (average patient age, 65 years); the survival rate at 12 years was 93%.[1] An additional cobalt-chrome metal-backed support has been used since 1984 (Mod III knee) (Richards, Smith & Nephew) to improve the mechanical properties of the implant and thereby increase the indications for unicondylar arthroplasty (UCA) in middle-aged patients. The failure rate at 10-year follow-up was abnormally high, primarily because of loosening from early polyethylene wear.

These findings led to the design in 1991 of the Genesis Uni prosthesis (Smith & Nephew), consisting of a 2-mm titanium metal-backed support with optional screw fixation, which may be used with or without cement, and an adjustable polyethylene insert. The second option is a full polyethylene tibial plateau that, unlike the Marmor implant, allows for a complete cortical rim support.

One or more of the authors or the departments with which they are affiliated have received something of value from a commercial or other party related directly or indirectly to the subject of this chapter.

Materials and Methods

Only 2 of 96 Genesis Uni prostheses implanted in middle-aged patients have been lost to follow-up. This series, therefore, contains 94 prostheses that were implanted in 91 patients (3 bilateral). Of the implants, 57 were metal-backed (13 cementless) and 37 were all polyethylene. The 47 men and 44 women in the series underwent 70 medial and 24 lateral arthroplasties. Average patient age at the time of surgery was 50 years (range, 24 to 60 years). The average follow-up period was 7 years 6 months (range, 5 to 10 years). The main etiologies were primary osteoarthritis (57), secondary osteoarthritis (28), osteonecrosis (5), and others (4).

Results

The Knee Society rating system was used to grade results. The knee score was 47.43 preoperatively and 94 postoperatively. No significant difference was noted between the medial (93.43) and lateral (94.44) UCAs; however, men (96.51) scored higher than women (91.36). The function score was 48.68 preoperatively and 94.43 postoperatively, with the lateral UCA (95.53) scoring slightly higher than the medial (93.53), and again, men (97.49) scored higher than women (92.05).

The absence of any significant overall difference between knee and function scores in this series can be attributed to the relatively young patient age. Patients in this age group typically do not present with other notable associated articular or spinal pathologies. No residual

FIGURE 1

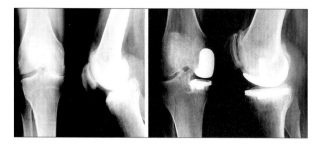

Moderate polyethylene wear at 10 years' follow-up in a 51-year-old man.

patellofemoral problems were observed. A lateral release was systematically performed in patients undergoing lateral UCAs and in half of those undergoing medial UCAs.

All of the patients involved in intense, work-related physical activity (eg, farmers, builders, laborers) returned to work. Nineteen of the patients participated in a noncontact sport before the articular disease and were able to resume activity at the preoperative level.

Complications

Five patients experienced complications. Cemented metal-backed tibial plateaus loosened in two patients who had undergone numerous operations and presented with underlying bone of poor quality. UCA was preferred to total knee arthroplasty (TKA) in these patients because of their age. The other complications were posttraumatic loosening of a metal-backed prosthesis, varus femorotibial instability that appeared progressively in a highly active patient with a full polyethylene medial UCA, and persistent pain syndrome with weight bearing in a patient with a cementless screwed metal-backed prosthesis with screw implantation. Revisions, including insertion of three mobile bearing TKAs and exchange of two unicondylar prostheses, had no negative effects.

Radiographic Results

The study of the positioning of the implants did not reveal any notable anomalies. The need for a slight safety under-correction to protect the healthy compartment, which has always appeared necessary for UCA, has been respected.[2] The average postoperative alignment for the medial arthroplasties was 2.5° of mechanical varus. The alignment for the lateral arthroplasties was 4° of mechanical valgus. No deterioration has been observed at the level of the healthy compartment or of the patellofemoral joint.

The average polyethylene wear was 0.5 mm (Figure 1). Significant wear of more than 1 mm was observed in three patients (two obese and one high-level tennis player) at 8 years' follow-up.

BENEFITS OF UNICONDYLAR ARTHROPLASTY

The decision to perform UCA is made only after the failure of the usual conservative rheumatologic, physiotherapeutic, and sometimes arthroscopic procedures. Therefore, the benefits of this procedure must be established in comparison with the two other choices–high tibial osteotomy (HTO) and TKA.

Benefits of UCA Versus HTO

The choice between HTO and UCA must be carefully considered. Obviously, there is no question of replacing an HTO with a UCA in elective surgery on patients younger than age 60 years. However, if an HTO is contraindicated, it should not be used in place of a UCA only because the patient is too young for an implant. Some of these inappropriate HTOs produce anatomic conditions that make it impossible to propose a modular replacement when rapid failure occurs in patients who are still young. The only solution at this stage is to carry out a TKA with bone and, sometimes, ligament sacrifice, which does not provide the resurfacing advantages of the UCA, which is the opposite of a half total knee.[3] The typical contraindications of HTO that should lead to UCA are described below.

Loss of Over 50% of Joint Space

In this situation, which is highlighted on weight-bearing long-leg radiographs and is confirmed by AP views at 20° flexion, HTO serves only to slow the progression of the arthrosis. The pain is not completely eliminated, and most patients must undergo revision with a TKA within a shorter timeframe than patients who have osteotomies when their loss of joint space is less than 50%.

Lootvoet and associates[4] studied the effects on outcome of the amount of joint space lost on a series of 193 closed-wedge valgus osteotomies. At 5 years' follow-up, satisfactory results were reported in 84% of patients when the initial narrowing of the medial joint line was less than 50%, and satisfactory results were reported in 60% when initial narrowing was more than 50%.

Monocompartmental Wear Without Any Tibial Bow (Straight Tibia)

An HTO may relieve the excessive stress on a subjacent compartment above a diaphyseal bow while conserving a horizontal joint line. However, the same does not apply where there is monocompartmental deterioration above a straight tibia in a patient whose lack of authentic physical tibial bow has been confirmed by weight-bearing long-leg radiographs.

The cartilage deterioration in the latter case is of purely articular origin, frequently as a result of the sequelae of sometimes iterative meniscectomy, knee instability caused by patellar or ligament problems, or the long-standing presence of excess weight. In these patients, HTO induces an oblique joint line, the consequence of which is increased overload at the level of the pathologic compartment with rapid aggravation of mechanical stress pain. When revision is needed, the anatomic conditions generated by the oblique joint line in patients who are still young removes all possibility of recourse to unicompartmental surgery and requires revision by TKA (Figure 2).

Anteroposterior Femorotibial Subluxation

AP femorotibial subluxation can be seen on weight-bearing lateral radiographs with the knee extended as far as possible. An HTO cannot stop the progression of the AP tibial displacement, resulting in spread of the arthrosis and the femoropatellar repercussions. Once the ligamentous origin of this subluxation has been eliminated by MRI or arthroscopy, its etiology, established by studying the anterior cruciate ligament (ACL), must be specified.

These tibial subluxations may be anterior as a result of the bony wear gap, or posterior as a result of osteophytes on the spinal eminence and of the intercondylar notch pushing the tibia back. The removal of the osteophytes and the restoration of a congruent joint surface by a unicompartmental implant acting as a shoehorn is the only means of reducing the sagittal subluxation.

Lateral Compartment Wear Secondary to Femoral Condyle Dysplasia

The outcome of an HTO in this case is an oblique joint line, which is obviously contraindicated. The severity of the effects of femoral osteotomy leads me to prefer unicompartmental replacement for middle-aged patients. The use of thick condyles (7 mm) instead of the standard 4-mm condyles makes it possible to compensate for the anomaly at its origin and to avoid the shift from the oppo-

FIGURE 2

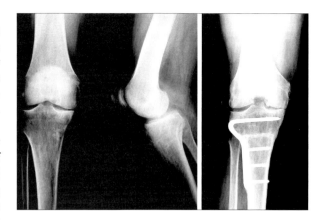

HTO failure at 7 years' follow-up for postmeniscectomy medial wear with a straight tibia.

site compartment that the use of a thicker tibial plateau would cause.

Posttraumatic Unicompartmental Osteoarthritis

In patients with posttraumatic sequelae in whom persistent tibial or femoral condyle depression has led to a localized posttraumatic osteoarthritic knee, the advantage of UCA is certain. This condition occurs after an insufficient attempt to surgically raise the condyle or an insufficient attempt to provide a solution for the extent of the cartilage damage. Contrary to the osteotomy, which corrects only the axial deviation, UCA allows the reestablishment of an anatomic articular congruence.

Failure of Previous High Tibial Osteotomy as a Result of Undercorrection

Failure of an HTO as a result of undercorrection must not lead to the simplistic reasoning that TKA is the only conceivable solution. TKA is a rather unattractive alternative, particularly for active patients younger than age 60 years.

When the extent of cartilage wear does not permit the use of another HTO to reestablish the correction of the axial deviation, UCA makes it possible, subject to the integrity of the ACL, to obtain the same quality of result as with a primary procedure. However, the results of UCA are unfavorable when it is used for a recurrence of the unicompartmental damage caused by the failure of a neutrally aligned or overcorrected HTO.[5]

FIGURE 3

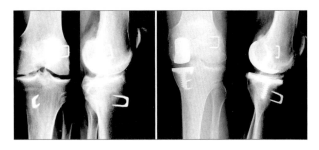

Unicondylar knee and ACL reconstruction in a 44-year-old physical education teacher at 10 years' follow-up.

Benefits of UCA Versus TKA

Obviously, UCA is not more beneficial than TKA where the arthrosis involves the two femorotibial compartments or combines femoropatellar deterioration with limited unicompartmental lesions. It is, however, surprising to see that most surgeons, particularly in the United States, continue to favor TKA when the extent of the isolated unicompartmental lesions no longer allows consideration of an HTO. The arguments used to support TKA do not really seem to be confirmed by qualitative elements in the light of the results presented at the beginning of this study and in other long-term series.[6-8] The advantages of UCA compared with TKA are, however, indisputable.

Preservation of Soft Tissues

The preservation of soft tissues represents the most important advantage of UCA. The absence of medial, lateral, or posterior release and conservation of the ACL allow normal proprioception of the knee to be restored, which occurs only exceptionally when the knee is fitted with total implants. The other advantage of respecting the ACL, as shown in biomechanical studies,[9] is the reestablishment of a normal gait pattern.

Chassin and associates[10] reported the adduction moment patterns for knees of normal subjects, patients with UCA, and patients with TKA. The adduction moment pattern in all patients with UCA was identical to that found in normal subjects; this was not true for patients with TKA. These authors believe that the essential difference in the functional results between the two types of knee replacement is directly related to the conservation of the ACL. It should be noted that in our series,[1] patients with severe unicompartmental arthrosis secondary to an instability of the ACL have undergone associ-

ated ACL reconstruction: five before the UCA (Figure 3), four at the same time, and one 4 months later.

The functional results obtained in patients judged to be too young or to have too demanding a level of physical activity to consider a TKA appeared identical to those obtained in patients who initially had the classic indications for UCA.

Mini-Invasive Technique

The mini-invasive technique initially described by Repicci (see chapter 8), whose long-term results recently have been reported,[11] represents a major advantage compared with TKA. It has a faster recovery time, shorter hospital stay, and a limited incision without everting the patella. The recent attempts at mini-invasive TKA have found the procedure to be much more delicate than UCA because of the space taken up by the trial implants and jigs and of the risk of patellar tendon avulsion.

The main disadvantage of the mini-invasive procedure, although the most recent instrumentation is accurate, is that it does not provide a sufficiently good view of the surgical site without resection of a part of the patellar facet corresponding to the approach. I do not perform this resection on the medial side because it causes a problem with the positioning of the patellar button in cases of revision. The risk of the resulting poorer view is a return to the failures of the past that caused the bad reputation of UCA.

Visual inspection of the perioperative trial insertion of the prostheses before cementing them is the best guarantee of the quality of their positioning and is indispensable to obtain a valid future result. At present, it is still too early for computer-assisted surgery to be able to guarantee proper positioning. Therefore, I prefer the less invasive arthroplasty procedure that, while respecting the patella, extends the incision medially or laterally by two or three fingerwidths at the suprapatellar muscle level.

If the patella is not everted and when the suprapatellar pouch is respected, this technique, which allows a decent view, leads to the same faster recovery time and shorter hospital stay as the stricter mini-invasive technique proposed by Repicci (see chapter 8). My ongoing double-blind study of the speed of recovery after the two procedures has not revealed any differences.

Greater Mobility

The UCA provides greater mobility than the average for TKAs: 120° in my series of middle-aged patients penalized by posttraumatic sequelae, compared with the 126° in the initial series of Marmor prostheses presented in 1996.[1] This type of result can be obtained only when TKA is carried out by an extensive release of the soft tissues, particularly the posterior cruciate ligament, with at worst the risk of instability and at best the formal loss of proprioception inherent to this procedure.

Cost

The cost of UCA is much more reasonable both at the research level and at the implant level. This obvious fact, already illustrated by Bonnutti and Kester,[12] appears all the more topical in the context of the current negative economic situation of most international health care systems.

Greater Ease of Revision

UCA is easier to revise in cases of failure than for TKA, which may appear surprising given the negative opinions expressed on this subject.[13] The difficulties of revision mentioned by the different authors have appeared to be absolutely unfounded in light of the 22 knees out of a series of 944 Genesis Uni prosthesis operations I have performed since 1991, regardless of patient age.[14] The main reasons for this absence of difficulty in the revisions are the use of resurfacing femoral implants, the use of a minimum quantity of cement on the tibia, and annual radiologic follow-up.

Apart from the posterior resection, which has no future consequences in cases of revision, the prosthetic condyle must rest on the underlying subchondral bone whose mechanical resistance (being much higher than that of the cancellous bone) protects against loosening. Loosening has occurred in only one patient with posttraumatic origin in the Genesis resurfacing femoral implant series[2] and in two patients with medial condyle osteonecrosis in the Marmor series.[1] The use of a small quantity of cement is a fundamental factor in facilitating revision. Invasive cementing, particularly at the tibial level, does not improve the quality of fixation of the implant and can only complicate the revision as a result of the existence of a cavitary defect requiring complementary bone grafting. The autostability of the trial template without any tilting during the full range of motion from 0° to 130° of flexion represents a more formal guarantee of its long-term fixation than excessive cementing.[14]

In highly active male patients, the solution that is chosen more and more often and that is borne out by the

work of Epinette and Edidin[15] is the use of a cementless screwed plateau with a hydroxyapatite coating that allows bone ingrowth fixation. This type of implant allows a high level of activity with no worry about loosening. At the femoral level, revision is facilitated by the absence of cementing at the level of the central peg hole.

Annual radiologic follow-up provides a backup that contributes to the simplicity of the revision. In UCA, tibial loosening remains asymptomatic for a long period, and the patient frequently comes back too late, at the sinkage stage. Therefore, I recommend annual follow-up for unicompartmental prostheses, even in the absence of any clinical symptoms.

PITFALLS OF UNICOMPARTMENTAL ARTHROPLASTY

Most of the pitfalls of UCA have a technical origin because this procedure is more technically demanding than TKA. The pitfalls are different for valgus and varus deviation. In varus deviation, the most commonly observed mistakes are incorrect tibial resection in the frontal plane, overcorrection, and excessive lateral laxity. In valgus deviation, the most commonly observed pitfalls are secondary subluxation caused by incorrect centering between the femoral and tibial components and excessive undercorrection.

Tibial Resection in the Frontal Plane

If there is a bony varus deformity of the tibia, the cut must be at right angles to the epiphyseal axis rather than to the mechanical axis of the tibia, as for a TKA. If this is not done, the inevitable result will be a progressive frontal femorotibial subluxation, leading to painful contact between the prosthetic condyle and the spinal eminence and to femorotibial instability in a weight-bearing situation. To avoid this mistake, the angle of the tibial cut must be calculated preoperatively and be transferred to the pretibial jig, which is adapted to a horizontal mobile plateau including a goniometer (Figure 4).

Overcorrection

There is a major risk of overcorrection with deterioration of the healthy compartment and a bony varus deformity being turned in a valgus one. Overcorrection is the main cause of the failures observed in the first series of unicompartmental implants in which the essential criterion

FIGURE 4

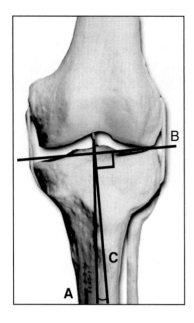

Cartier angle. A, Tibial mechanical axis (center of the knee to the middle of the ankle). B, Line tangential to the lateral tibial plateau. C, Line perpendicular to line B.

advocated by Marmor,[16] the undercorrection of the knee, was not followed. This philosophy differs radically from the principles underlying osteotomies and TKA. The UCA needs only to fill the gap of the bone loss without correcting the varus bow. Anatomic perioperative landmarks for undercorrection must be followed; the most important of these is a slight remaining laxity of the medial side at 15° of flexion without any laxity in extension.[14]

Excessive Lateral Laxity

This parameter must be checked during trials when the area with arthritic loss of bone stock, which may mimic laxity in the opposite compartment, is filled with the trial component. If, when applying a stress on the convex side with the knee slightly flexed (as in the weight-bearing situation of walking), there is sliding, with the trial condyle coming into contact with the spinal eminence. This proves that there is true ligamentous laxity of the convex side and indicates the need for TKA. This test obviously is valid only if the orientation of the tibial cut has met the criteria established previously.

Before carrying out all the prosthetic trials, it is impossible to guarantee that the indication for UCA can be maintained. Therefore, UCA is done subject to the availability of a patellar tendon graft during the operation and the possibility of fixation with or without cement.

Cementless fixation is preferred whenever it is feasible in active, middle-aged male patients.

Problems With Femorotibial Centering

In many valgus knees, ideal condyle centering in flexion will result in an overmedialized trial condyle in extension that is really too close to or even in contact with the spinal eminence. A deliberately laterally off-center positioning of the trial condyle is necessary to achieve anatomic alignment between the condyle and the tibial plateau in extension and during normal walking. For this reason, the lateral condylar osteophyte on which the implant can easily be rested is left in place.

This peculiarity of adjustment explains the difference between external lateral mobile unicondylar knee arthroplasties and those practiced at medial compartment level as illustrated by Goodfellow and O'Connor.[17] The most probable explanation of this phenomenon is that in the valgus knee the prostheses are placed on a knee in external subluxation, which must not be corrected by the implant. Any attempt to correct the external subluxation would require lateral soft-tissue tightening by excessively thick prosthetic shims that could only cause an overload at the level of the healthy compartment, with secondary degenerative changes caused by an overcorrection.

Excessive Undercorrection

In the case of significant lateral condyle dysplasia, I favor a thick femoral component (7 mm) rather than the standard 4-mm component. This compensation by thick condyle allows the correction of not only the inferior but also the posterior condyle dysplasia. The stabilization that the thick condyle affords is better than compensation at the tibial level because it avoids articular shift in relation to the healthy compartment and limits the risk of later loss of correction.

CONCLUSION

In cases of degenerative arthritis in active middle-aged patients, UCA should override HTO contraindications and be selected over TKA every time the ACL is functional and the opposite tibial and femoropatellar compartments are preserved.

The causes of the poor reputation of these implants that has led to their discredit, especially in the United States, have been analyzed over time. Recently, renewed interest in this procedure has resulted in closer analysis of the results. These causes include poor technique, poor implant design, insufficient polyethylene thickness, too rigid metal-backed supports (cobalt chrome), and, for many years, an inappropriate sterilization process corresponding to the period of use of gamma radiation. Inappropriate patient or implant selection should also be stressed and remains a problem that has not been completely resolved—in particular the choice between an implant with a metal-backed support and one that is all polyethylene.

Subject to meeting the need for thorough training in knee implants in specialized centers in order to achieve the learning curve that is much more demanding than for TKA and to having sufficient experience in knee surgery to maintain and improve the surgeon's personal practice, the return of this procedure can only be beneficial, especially for middle-aged patients.

References

1. Cartier P, Sanouiller JL, Grelsamer RP: Unicompartmental knee arthroplasty surgery: 10 years minimum follow-up period. *J Arthroplasty* 1996;11,7:782-788.

2 Cartier P, Cheaib S: Unicondylar knee arthroplasty 2-10 years of follow-up evaluation. *J Arthroplasty* 1987;2:157-162.

3. Grelsamer RP, Cartier P: A unicompartmental knee replacement is not "half a total knee": Five major differences. *Orthop Rev* 1992;21:1350-1356.

4. Lootvoet L, Massinon A, Rossillon R, Himer O, Lambert K: Ghosez JP: Ostéotomie tibiale haute de valgisation pour gonarthrose sur genu varum: A propos d'une série de cent quatre-vingt treize cas revus après 6 à 10 ans de recul. *Rev Chir Orthop* 1993;79:375-384

5. Cartier P, Sanouiller JL: La prothèse unicompartimentale du genou dans les échecs d'ostéotomie tibiale de valgisation pour gonarthrose: A propos de 25 cas. *Rev Chir Orthop Reparatrice Appar Mot* 1992;78:112-114.

6. Scott RD, Cobb AG, McQueary FG, Thornhill TS: Unicompartmental knee arthroplasty: Eight- to 12-year fol-low-up evaluation with survivorship analysis. *Clin Orthop* 1991;271:96-100.

7. Capra SW Jr, Fehring TK: Unicondylar arthroplasty: A survivorship analysis. *J Arthroplasty* 1992;7:247-251.

8. Bergmann EG: Süssenbach F: The unicondylar knee replacement as a treatment of varus/valgus osteoarthritis of the knee: Middle and long term results, in Cartier P, Epinette JA, Deschamps G, Hernigou P (eds): *Unicompartmental Knee Arthroplasty*. Paris, France, Expansion Scientifique Française, 1997, pp 180–191.

9. Bensadoun SL: Biomechanical aspect of unicompartmental arthroplasty, in Cartier P, Epinette JA, Deschamps G, Hernigou P (eds): *Unicompartmental Knee Arthroplasty*. Paris, France, Expansion Scientifique Française, 1997, pp 3-11.

10. Chassin EP, Mikosz RP, Andriacchi TP, Rosenberg AG: Functional analysis of cemented medial unicompartmental knee arthroplasty. *J Arthroplasty* 1996;5:553-559.

11. Romanowski MR, Repicci JA: Minimally invasive unicondylar arthroplasty: Eight years follow-up. *J Knee Surg* 2002;15:17-22.

12. Bonutti PM, Kester MA: Unicompartmental knee arthroplasty: A US experience; in Cartier P, Epinette JA, Deschamps G, Hernigou P (eds): *Unicompartmental Knee Arthroplasty.* Paris, France, Expansion Scientifique Française 1997, pp 261-266.

13. Padgett DE, Stern SH, Insall JN: Revision total knee arthroplasty for failed unicompartmental replacement. *J Bone Joint Surg Am* 1991;73:186-190.

14. Cartier Ph: Unicompartmental prosthetic replacement, in *Surgical Techniques in Orthopaedics and Traumatology.* Paris, France, Editions Scientifiques et Médicales Elsevier SAS, 2000,55-570-A-10.

15. Epinette JA, Edidin AA: Hydroxyapatite coated unicompartmental knee replacement: A report of five to six years follow-up of the H.A. Unix tibial component, in Cartier P, Epinette JA, Deschamps G, Hernigou P (eds): *Unicompartmental Knee Arthroplasty*. Paris, France, Expansion Scientifique Française, 1997, pp 243–260.

16. Marmor L: The modular (Marmor) knee: Case report with a follow-up of 2 years. *Clin Orthop* 1976;120:86-94.

17. Goodfellow J, O'Connor JJ: The anterior cruciate ligament in knee arthroplasty: A risk-factor with unconstrained meniscal prostheses. *Clin Orthop* 1990;276:245-252.

CHAPTER *8*

UNICONDYLAR KNEE REPLACEMENT: THE AMERICAN EXPERIENCE

JOHN A. REPICCI, MD
JODI F. HARTMAN, MS

Prior to the mid 1900s, no viable surgical reconstruction options for the treatment of sclerotic-stage osteoarthritis (OA) of the knee existed. The MacIntonish and McKeever metallic spacers, developed during the late 1950s and early 1960s, were important early innovations in knee arthroplasty.[1] Significant progress regarding the development of knee prostheses occurred in the 1970s.[1] Although most of the prostheses designed during this time are no longer in use, many of the concepts have been applied to modern designs; these designs may be classified as either constrained or surface-replacement prostheses. The constrained prostheses are hinged, whereas the surface replacement prostheses have either bicondylar or unicondylar designs. Bicondylar, or total knee arthroplasty (TKA), prostheses are considered true total joint replacement devices and involve the replacement of both femorotibial compartments and, typically, the patellofemoral compartment. In addition, these prostheses require a certain degree of ligamentous balancing, which may be addressed by retaining, excising, or substituting the posterior cruciate ligament.

Unicondylar, or unicondylar knee arthroplasty (UKA), prostheses are segmental replacement devices designed to replace only the affected tibiofemoral compartment, leaving the remainder of the joint. Unicondylar devices may be categorized into the following classes: (1) resurfacing designs, which use bone-sparing resurfacing components and were introduced and developed in the early 1970s;[2] (2) resection designs, which involve resections and instrumentation similar to that of TKA; and (3) mobile bearing designs, which were originally developed in 1978[3] with the goals of achieving more physiologic knee kinematics and offering maximal conformity between the articulating components with minimum constraint. The design concepts of each type of UKA and the surgical technique for its implantation will be discussed later in this chapter.

In 1972, Marmor[2] introduced an unconstrained UKA device designed to resurface the arthritic knee joint with minimal bone loss. This resurfacing device permits normal rotation of the knee joint with a true polycentric femoral component and allows replacement of either one or both tibiofemoral compartments, relying on the ligaments for inherent stability.[2,4] Bone preservation is achieved by both the resurfacing technique and the ability to independently replace either tibiofemoral compartment when only one is affected. The potential benefits of this conservative approach include minimal bone resection, which does not compromise possible future revision, and decreased surgical morbidity.[4] Marmor's pioneering development and the promising initial results of his design as a single-compartment knee replacement device[2,4] launched the concept of using UKA for the treatment of unicompartmental OA.

Throughout the 1970s and 1980s, orthopaedic surgeons continued developing and using UKA designs. Although many authors reported positive results with UKA,[5-7] high failure rates began to emerge,[8-10] especially within the United States. Disappointing results of a resection UKA design led Insall and Aglietti[8] to abandon the use of UKA for the treatment of medial unicompartmental OA, recommending either tibial osteotomy or TKA instead. However, good results led Insall and Walker[9] to conclude that UKA was a viable treatment option for lateral unicompartmental OA, a condition that was not successfully treated by tibial osteotomy; they stipulated, however, that this was the only indication for UKA.[8] Insall's studies[8,9] in particular seemed to affect the treatment trends in the United States, and use of UKA began to decline.[6]

Coinciding with the contradictory reports of UKA success, TKA use was increasing because of the technological advances of the 1980s, specifically improvements in polyethylene quality, enhanced surgical instrumentation, and better surgical techniques. As a result of the various unsatisfactory reports of UKA and the favorable reports of TKA,[11-13] many surgeons, predominantly those in the United States, abandoned use of the UKA. By the early 1990s, TKA was well recognized as the ultimate salvage procedure and soon became the standard to which all other knee procedures were compared.

However, UKA remained a viable treatment option for unicompartmental OA in Europe throughout the 1980s and early 1990s. European surgeons and a few surgeons from the United States (including the senior author, John Repicci) remained dedicated to the continued development of UKA. A better understanding of the biomechanics and modes of failure of the early UKA devices led to improvement of the original UKA designs. The design of special instrumentation, the development of better patient selection criteria, and, perhaps above all, the addition of a minimally invasive surgical technique,[14] contributed to the low morbidity and rapid rehabilitation of UKA—the hallmarks of the procedure that once were recognized as advantages.

These advances and the continued use of UKA by others laid the groundwork for its recent revival in the United States.[15-21] The use of UKA in the United States continues to increase as more surgeons learn of its low morbidity and rapid rehabilitation of patients. It must be stressed, however, that the resurgence in UKA is, in part, a response by orthopaedic surgeons to meet patient demand. The conservative nature of the procedure, combined with the low morbidity, rapid rehabilitation, and desirable level of postoperative function, appeals to many patients with unicompartmental OA of the knee who, after learning about the procedure through word-of-mouth or various media sources, often approach orthopaedic surgeons requesting UKA.

LESSONS LEARNED FROM FIRST-GENERATION DESIGNS

In retrospect, most of the original UKA failures were a result of design problems, errors in surgical technique, and/or improper patient selection.[6,8,22-25] Constrained designs with a groove or track limited the rotation of the replaced compartment, compared with normal rotation in the contralateral compartment, subjecting the device to increased stress, which ultimately led to increased polyethylene wear, tibial loosening, and subsequent failure.[26] Many early UKA prostheses with blunt anterior femoral edges impinged on the patella and subsequently failed.[26] In addition, the common use of a thin 6-mm polyethylene tibial component resulted in early loosening and failure due to deformity.[3,6,10,26-28] Metal-backed tibial components were introduced in an attempt to address the deformity issue, but the thin layer of polyethylene often led to polyethylene wear-through.[3,29]

Because of the learning curve associated with use of UKA, many technical mistakes made during this initial period were the result of surgeon inexperience.[6,16,23,30] Although UKA prostheses may be relatively easy to insert, accurate component alignment and positioning, along with attention to soft-tissue integrity and balancing, are of utmost importance.[8,25] One common mistake in the early use of UKA was the use of an excessively thick tibial component to intentionally overcorrect the knee joint.[9] This practice converted former varus deformities into valgus deformities, which overloaded both the tibial component and the unaffected compartment, resulting in contralateral compartment degeneration, polyethylene wear, and subsequent UKA failure.[3,10,17,23,26,28,31,32] The use of an excessively thick tibial component also explains why many early UKA failures occurred with medial compartment devices, whereas lateral compartment UKA often was successful.[8-10] Avoiding overcorrection has greatly reduced the incidence of UKA failures in recent years.[5,15,17,27,31]

Finally, lack of well-established selection criteria resulted in implantation in some patients who, in hindsight, were not proper candidates for UKA. More specifically, UKA initially was used not only for unicompartmental OA but also for diseases and conditions, such as rheumatoid arthritis and gross instability, that are common contraindications according to today's criteria.[4,15,17,22,31-33] In conclusion, preliminary UKA designs, coupled with errors in surgical technique and improper patient selection, were responsible for most of the failures reported in the 1970s and early 1980s. The ensuing complications and unsatisfactory survivorship contributed to the reduction in the number of UKAs performed in the United States.

ADVANCES IN SECOND-GENERATION DESIGNS

Many of the UKA systems currently available in the United States are improved versions of the original resurfacing, resection, and mobile bearing designs. These UKA systems differ in design and in the surgical techniques required for implantation. The improvements, strengths, and weaknesses of each are discussed below.

Resurfacing Designs

Versions of the original Marmor design remain in use today. Although the Marmor prosthesis is well proven, as indicated by successful results obtained by nondesigning surgeons,[27,30,32,34,35] attempts have been made to further enhance it. The Repicci II Unicondylar Knee System (Biomet, Inc, Warsaw, IN) is based on the original Marmor design, with two modifications: (1) the femoral component has been rounded medially and laterally to decrease edge wear, and (2) the articulating surface of the tibial component has been slightly contoured to better conform to the femoral component. These adjustments also allow the use of a tibial component with a decreased thickness compared with Marmor's design.

Resurfacing UKA designs incorporate inlay tibial and femoral components, use a resurfacing surgical technique, and have an anatomic basis. Previous studies of the progression of OA of the knee have indicated that OA is a slow, progressive disease, typically limited to one tibiofemoral compartment and predominately beginning in the medial compartment.[36,37] As OA develops, the body compensates for articular cartilage loss by forming sclerotic bone at the medial tibia. This bone assists the medial compartment in withstanding joint loading, supporting

weight, and permitting continued ambulation for 10 to 18 years after initiation of the disease.[37] This sclerotic medial tibia, also referred to as the medial tibial buttress, is broader and thicker than a normal tibia. Resurfacing designs use the medial tibial buttress for support of the inlay tibial components. Because medial tibial bone loss has been cited as a major problem in converting UKA to TKA,[22,38] a major advantage of using an all-polyethylene inlay tibial component is that minimal bone resection is required, which preserves the medial tibial buttress. Thus, the bone-preserving nature of the resurfacing technique and the design of the inlay components increase the likelihood that future conversion to TKA may be accomplished easily without significant bone loss.

The two main disadvantages underscored by opponents of resurfacing UKA designs are the same as the advantages highlighted by its advocates. Issues of accuracy and reproducibility have been raised regarding the freehand resurfacing technique in which alignment is achieved without the use of instrumentation guides.[19,33] However, recent improvements in instrumentation, such as the use of rapid reaming systems, have alleviated some of this criticism[35] and, with proper surgeon training and expertise, such errors should not be a concern. The remaining disadvantage cited is the use of sclerotic bone as support for the tibial component. Although resurfacing advocates recognize that the formation of the medial tibial buttress is not an efficient process and acknowledge that the quality of subsequent bone is not superior compared with subchondral bone, they prefer to use this supplemental sclerotic bone rather than resecting precious subchondral bone, as is done in resection and mobile bearing UKA. According to Grelsamer,[31] the design of certain implants requires more bone removal than others. Greater problems, which often necessitate bone grafting, arise at revision if osseous collapse involves the tibial cortical rim, a situation less likely to arise with Marmor-type tibial implants.[31] Therefore, resurfacing UKA is advantageous not only because it incorporates the use of the medial tibial buttress without resecting valuable bone stock but also because it is minimally invasive and is capable of extending the spectrum of knee survivability by approximately 10 years without detrimentally affecting potential future revision surgery.

Survivorship of 90% or greater at a minimum follow-up of 10 years for resurfacing designs has been reported by nondesigning surgeons,[27,32] with one study reporting a 22-year survivorship of 93%, defined by revision due to aseptic loosening, at a minimum follow-up of 15 years.[32] A 4% revision rate requiring conversion to TKA among Ahlback stage 2 and 3 patients at 8 years has been reported by Romanowski and Repicci.[39]

Resection Designs

Current UKA resection designs integrate modular saw-cut components with a resection technique similar to that used in TKA, and most include jig-type guide instrumentation to assist in proper insertion of the components. The main modifications of second-generation resection UKA designs are the use of thicker all-polyethylene tibial components and the addition of metal-backed tibial components.[15,28]

The major advantages of resection UKA designs are related to surgical technique and the associated instrumentation. The similarity between the resections performed in UKA and TKA may offer some degree of technical familiarity to orthopaedic surgeons who routinely perform TKA. In addition, the use of instrumentation in resection UKA provides a standardized method of inserting components, which may assist in ensuring proper component alignment and orientation.[33] According to Bert,[33] proper instrumentation allows for more precise anatomic resections that result in better component fit, a more normal femorotibial angle, and less bone resection than performing the technique freehand. Many UKA failures have occurred as a result of improper component positioning that, in turn, often was attributable to poor instrumentation.[19] Consequently, advocates of instrumentation use in conjunction with UKA contend that inserting components without instrumentation is inaccurate.[19,33] Laskin[19] further asserts that instrumentation use is critical and that components inserted by eye alone cannot be expected to function well.

Even when instrumentation is used, a significant shortcoming of resection UKA is the high degree of surgical skill and experience required to perform this technically demanding procedure. As discussed previously, a learning curve is associated with UKA,[3,6,16,23,30,35,40] and the surgical technique is different than that of TKA.[18,31] Moreover, resection UKA designs may require more surgical accuracy than resurfacing designs to avoid malpositioning and malalignment.[25] These technical errors may result from the significant tibial and femoral resections involved with resection UKA, which may lead to increased contact stress and subsequent wear of the polyethylene tibial component.[25,30,34] The poor results of several resection UKA

designs have led Knutson and associates[34] to conclude that their survivorship is inferior to that of traditional resurfacing designs.

Moreover, as demonstrated by several Swedish Knee Registry studies,[25,34,41] instrumentation in and of itself neither negates surgical skill nor improves survivability. Knutson and associates[41] found the revision rate of several newer jig-type resection designs to be approximately two times higher than that of the traditional resurfacing designs. Although they acknowledged that the higher revision rate may be due to a learning curve, the authors questioned whether it was inherent to the resection UKA designs and questioned the supposed advantage of using such jig-type designs. Even with the use of guide instrumentation to assist in maintaining the parallel positioning of the components in extension and in flexion, surgical skill remains particularly important in resection UKA.[25] A primary difference between resection and resurfacing designs is that the femoral component in resurfacing designs has a constant radius, which may explain why it is less likely to fail earlier than the resection designs.[25] Another reason that guide instrumentation does not "save the day" when used in conjunction with resection UKA involves the nature of unicompartmental medial OA, also referred to as "extension gap disease" (Figure 1). Although the guide instrumentation used with resection UKA designs aids in producing accurate resections, it does not address ligament balance, which is crucial in ensuring a successful outcome, regardless of design. If soft-tissue balancing is not addressed in addition to performing the proper resections, the likelihood of producing a successful outcome is greatly diminished.

The foremost disadvantage of properly performed resection UKA is the significant amount of bone loss, which may complicate potential future conversion to TKA. Resection UKA involves the removal of significantly more bone than resurfacing UKA and, if jig instrumentation is used, often requires full exposure of the joint. In addition, because modular resection tibial components are much thicker and wider than their resurfacing counterparts, the medial tibial buttress must be sacrificed. Because the joint line of the uninvolved compartment is not altered in unicompartmental OA, elevation of the joint line with a thick tibial component is not an option in UKA.[37] Therefore, the thick tibial components incorporated into resurfacing UKA designs require a considerable amount of tibial bone resection. The use of pegs or fins, common fixation methods in resection UKA, further compromises tibial bone

FIGURE 1

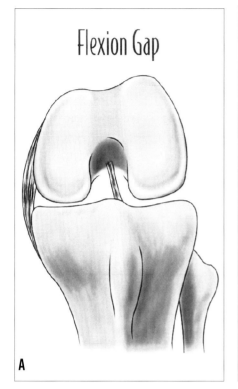

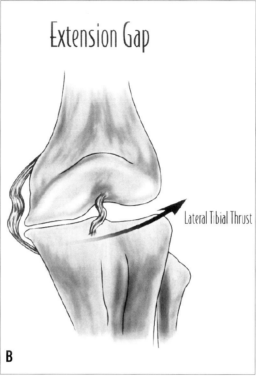

Unicompartmental medial OA is an extension gap disease. **A,** Unicompartmental medial OA does not affect the flexion gap and, consequently, there is no associated loss of articular surface or deformity. **B,** This disease affects the extension gap and produces approximately 5 mm of articular space loss, which causes several ramifications, including ACL and medial collateral ligament laxity, as well as lateral tibial thrust, or varus deformity, in the extension gap.

during component removal before revision surgery. Besides causing additional bone loss, these fixation devices further complicate revision surgery because bone grafts or special components, such as custom devices or metal-wedge tibial trays, often are required to stabilize the tibia.[21,22,28,38]

Finally, the studies commonly cited to corroborate the contention that UKA should not be performed because of the associated difficulties at revision due to medial tibial bone loss involve resection, not resurfacing, designs.[22,38] In a report of the results of 21 failed resection UKAs requiring revision to TKA, Padgett and associates[38] noted that the major osseous defects observed during revision were not surprising because of the large amount of tibial bone that was resected. They further concluded that it was difficult to justify the use of UKA on the basis that it conserves bone when a thick polyethylene tibial component, which is required in resection UKA prostheses, is used. It should be noted, however, that these revision studies involved the use of first-generation designs. Two more recent reports have suggested that revision of second-generation resection UKAs to TKA is straightforward and concluded that failed UKA may easily be converted to TKA.[20,24]

Highly specialized surgeons may produce excellent results with resection UKAs, as indicated by a multicenter study with 98% survivorship at 10 years.[15] However, surgeons performing too few UKAs per year may not acquire the expertise required to successfully perform these procedures.[25] This discrepancy between results substantiates that the survivorship of resection UKA prostheses is susceptible not only to patient selection and activity but also to technique, with a high degree of surgical skill and experience required to obtain successful results.[25] Therefore, it is of paramount importance for orthopaedic surgeons to realize that UKA is not "half a total knee"[18,31] and not to assume that the use of guide instrumentation makes the UKA technique similar to that of TKA and that it enhances UKA survivorship. The general orthopaedic surgeon population in the United States may or may not have the necessary experience with UKA and with ligament-balancing issues to obtain successful results. The recent trend of combining a minimally invasive surgical technique with UKA further increases the complexity of the procedure. Although the precise volume of resection UKAs required to establish and maintain the required surgical expertise is difficult to ascertain, it has been estimated that at least 10 to 15 UKAs per year are necessary to retain reasonable expertise.[25]

Mobile Bearing Designs

The first mobile bearing UKA design has undergone several modifications since its inception in 1978.[3] Because the original Oxford Meniscal prosthesis (Phase 1; Biomet, Ltd, Bridgend, Scotland) involved saw-cut femoral resections, precise ligament balancing was difficult to achieve, resulting in occasional subluxation of the mobile bearing.[42] In the mid 1980s, the initial femoral component with three flat internal facets fitted to angular saw-cut femoral resections was modified to a component with posteriorly flat and anteriorly spherically concave facets to fit a convex femoral surface prepared with a shaped bone mill.[42] The use of a bone mill with this phase II design permitted femoral resection in 1-mm increments, which assisted in obtaining accurate ligament balancing and subsequently decreased the incidence of mobile bearing dislocation.[42] In addition, an intramedullary jig was added to enhance femoral component alignment, and the anterior lip of the meniscal bearing was lowered by 1.5 mm to reduce the risk of impingement.[3] In 1998, further improvements in instrumentation and the addition of a minimally invasive surgical approach, which was first introduced in 1992,[14] resulted in a dramatic decrease in patient recovery time.[3] Using this minimally invasive approach with mobile bearing UKA resulted in recovery that was two times faster than after traditional UKA and three times faster than after TKA.[43,44]

The most significant advantage of mobile bearing designs versus other UKA designs may be reduced polyethylene wear.[3,25,45] Lindstrand and associates[25] noted that when the surgical technique is adequate, mobile bearing designs may exhibit less long-term polyethylene wear than resection designs. The Oxford design blends a spherical femoral component and a flat tibial component with an unconstrained mobile bearing that is spherically concave anteriorly and flat posteriorly.[42,45] The resulting combination is a fully congruent prosthesis that minimizes contact pressure and subsequent polyethylene wear.[42,45] A retrieval study of 16 medial UKA explants demonstrated an average penetration of 0.036 mm/yr and mean wear as

low as 0.01 mm/yr in the six devices precisely implanted with no evidence of impingement.[45] The unique design of mobile bearing UKA with its congruous articular surfaces maximizes contact area, which decreases contact stresses, and avoids excessive constraint, which results in more physiologic knee kinematics in both flexion and extension.[3,45]

Despite these notable advantages, the performance and survivorship of mobile bearing UKA are linked inextricably to the quality of its highly complex surgical procedure. Like resection UKAs, mobile bearing UKAs require a high degree of surgical accuracy to successfully implant the prosthesis.[3,17,42,45,46] The designing surgeons acknowledge this susceptibility to technical errors compared with other UKA designs, citing dependency of stability on ligament balancing as a possible explanation because it is an unconstrained design that is retained merely by its shape and soft-tissue tensioning.[3,42] Given the precise ligament balancing required and the mechanical complexity of mobile bearing UKA designs, proper implantation, avoiding possible impingement and subluxation, may be difficult to achieve because of the small margin of error.[3,45]

Another disadvantage of mobile bearing UKA designs is the significant femoral and tibial resections required for implantation of a three-component system, even when the thinnest mobile bearing is used. As is the case with resection UKA designs,[22,38] the substantial bone resection required for implantation, including sacrifice of the medial tibial buttress, may complicate potential future conversion to TKA. In addition, the polyethylene component of mobile bearing designs generally is thinner than its counterparts, theoretically placing the design at an increased risk of polyethylene wear and possible failure. However, polyethylene wear has not been cited as a common failure mode in mobile bearing UKA because of the high degree of conformity between the articulating components.[3,45-47] More frequently reported failure modes have included dislocation of the mobile bearing,[46,48] especially when implanted in the lateral compartment.[48]

A final drawback is that mobile bearing UKA designs are not available for widespread use in the United States. The US Food and Drug Administration (FDA) regulations require a minimum polyethylene thickness of 6 mm for implantation.[17] Thus, the Oxford Meniscal prosthesis, which is the original and perhaps most thoroughly researched mobile bearing UKA design, currently is not approved for use in the United States. It should be noted, therefore, that the designing surgeons of the Oxford, who advocate the use of mobile bearing designs and report excellent results,[3,42,44,45] are able to resect minimal bone while still using metal-backed tibial components because they operate outside the United States and are not restricted by FDA regulations.[17] Another design, the Low Contact Stress (LCS) mobile bearing knee system (DePuy; Warsaw, IN) has been approved by the FDA, and a newer version recently was released as the Preservation Minimally Invasive UKA System (DePuy). Compared with the Oxford design, a significant shortcoming of the LCS mobile bearing design is the dovetail track on the flat tibial portion of the device, which, in turn, transfers tremendous stress onto the curved femoral component, increasing the risk of femoral component loosening.

The results for implantation of mobile bearing UKA designs by designing surgeons are quite impressive.[3,42-44] Murray and associates[3] assert that patients with anteromedial OA and an intact ACL may be treated with a mobile bearing UKA instead of TKA without increasing the risk of failure in the first 10 years after implantation. The originators of the Oxford design have reported a survivorship of 98% at follow-up of 10 years.[3,42] However, results from the Swedish Knee Registry revealed that the skill required to implant mobile bearing UKA designs may not easily be transferred to the general orthopaedic population.[49] The findings from this study may explain the higher revision rate in Sweden compared with the low revision rates reported by the developers of the Oxford design.[3,42-44,46,49] Analysis by advocates of the Oxford design suggests that because the poor results obtained in the Swedish multicenter study occurred in only a few centers, these results demonstrate the learning curve associated with the procedure.[3,42,47] Consequently, the proponents of the Oxford design concluded that the discouraging results must be related to inappropriate technique and/or improper indications.[3,42,47] An outcome study by an independent center reported 2 revisions in 28 patients receiving an Oxford UKA implant (a 7.1% revision rate) who were not stringently selected and who were considered representative of the general total joint population.[40] In contrast, survivorship in other independent studies in which strict selection criteria were used is similar to that obtained by developers of the system,[47,50] with one report of a cumulative survival rate of 95% at 10 years under precise indications.[47] Clearly, research suggests that if mobile bearing UKA is performed by experienced surgeons and used in patients with early OA and ideal indications, a mobile bearing design may approach

the survivorship of TKA;[3,42,47,50] however, precision in surgical technique and patient selection is crucial.

REASONS FOR UNDERUTILIZATION OF UKA IN THE UNITED STATES

Statistics provide a striking contrast between use of UKA in the United States versus its use in Europe. According to the Swedish Arthroplasty Register,[40] UKA designs were used in approximately 30% of all knee arthroplasties reported in 1996 compared with only 5% of 250,000 knee arthroplasties performed in the United States in 1995. In contrast to the 250,000 TKAs performed in the United States in 1996 and 1997, only 2,500 UKAs were performed.[15] The underutilization of UKA in the United States is multifactorial.

The early disappointing UKA results reported by Americans in the late 1970s and early 1980s,[8-10] combined with the successful emergence of TKA,[11-13] certainly contributed to the minimal use of UKA in the United States throughout the 1980s.[6,15,18,40] Although based on obsolete first-generation designs, these reports, along with later negative reports on mediocre second-generation resection designs,[30,51] laid the foundation for the current preconceived perception that UKA is inferior to TKA.

As a result of this perception and/or because of the difficulty in teaching and learning proper UKA technique, UKA routinely is not taught in residency training programs in the United States. After departure from such programs, new surgeons are left with the impression that experienced surgeons prefer TKA over UKA and, because they observed satisfactory outcome of TKA during residency, many may conclude that TKA is better than its counterpart. The newly practicing surgeons continue using the familiar and reproducible TKA and, because many are general orthopaedic surgeons who perform a limited number of knee arthroplasties per year, may be less apt to perform UKA, a highly skilled procedure with a technique and instrumentation that may be unfamiliar.

Finally, at least in the past, less funding has been available for research and development of UKA designs versus TKA because most orthopaedic surgeons in the United States prefer TKA. From the time UKA fell out of favor in the United States in the 1980s, TKA has matured into a well-proven prosthetic procedure, whereas UKA remains a work in progress.

FIGURE 2

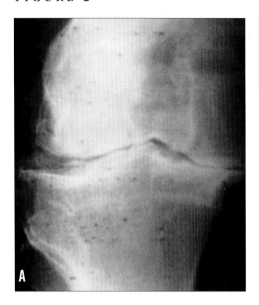 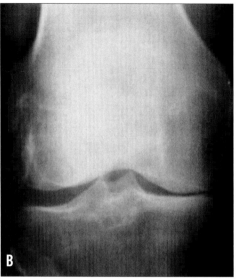

AP radiographs showing unicompartmental and tricompartmental OA. **A,** In tricompartmental OA, loss of both medial and lateral joint space occurs, with subluxation of the tibia in relation to the femur. **B,** In medial unicompartmental OA, narrowing or complete loss of medial joint space occurs, while the lateral joint space and medial tibial buttress are preserved.

THE INTRODUCTION OF A MINIMALLY INVASIVE APPROACH

By the early 1990s, TKA was well accepted as the ultimate knee salvage procedure in the United States. Alternative options for the treatment of unicompartmental OA that were in vogue at that time included arthroscopic débridement and high tibial osteotomy. Although popular, these treatments were not widely effective;[5,31,52-57] neither procedure addressed the pathology of OA, namely, loss of ligament balance and articular surface in the extension gap only.

During this time, Repicci recognized that knee osteoarthritis occurs in two common formats, tricompartmental and unicompartmental, each with a distinct clinical presentation (Figure 2). In tricompartmental OA, pain often is so debilitating that activities of daily living are severely restricted, independence is lost, and ambulatory aids, such as crutches, a walker, or a wheelchair, are required. If these patients desire pain relief and improved ambulation, TKA is the recommended surgical option due to the severity of disease progression. Fortunately, as previous studies examining the progression of knee OA have demonstrated, unicompartmental OA is far more prevalent than tricompartmental OA.[36,37] In unicompartmental OA, pain typically is inconvenient but not disabling. Because the disease and associated pain are not as severe,

patients with unicompartmental OA often are more active than those with tricompartmental OA. Consequently, such patients generally will not be satisfied with simple pain relief, but they may desire restored function and a return to activities of daily living. Because their OA is limited to a single tibiofemoral compartment, patients with unicompartmental OA are candidates for UKA and, when presented with a choice between UKA and TKA, tend to choose the less invasive procedure.[39]

Because UKA specifically focuses on the pathology of unicompartmental OA by combining realignment, replacement of a single damaged tibiofemoral compartment, and ligamentous balancing, Repicci believed that if some of the negative issues surrounding it were addressed, UKA would be a promising treatment option for a significant number of patients with unicompartmental OA. By using arthroscopy in conjunction with UKA, the morbidity of the procedure could be further reduced and the survivorship could be enhanced because arthroscopy would aid in excluding patients with advanced osteoarthritic involvement and/or a compromised meniscus in the contralateral compartment. Concerns regarding bone loss could be resolved by using a resurfacing UKA design, which uses sclerotic bone, preserves the medial tibial buttress, and, consequently, does not interfere with possible future conversion to TKA. In addition, the implementation of a multipronged program allowing UKA to be performed on an outpatient basis could further reduce the morbidity and cost associated with the procedure.

In 1999, Repicci and Eberle[14] reported on a minimally invasive UKA program begun by Repicci in 1992, combining arthroscopy, a minimally invasive surgical approach that emphasized avoiding patellar dislocation, resurfacing UKA, and pain management into a single program designed to avoid interference of physiology, lifestyle, and future treatment options. Prior to performing the UKA, arthroscopy is used to assess the articular cartilage of the contralateral compartment. Arthroscopy also allows examination of the contralateral meniscus, which is not visible by traditional exposure. Because the load-bearing surface area and stability of the knee are enhanced by intact menisci,[31,58-60] verification of a fully functional contralateral meniscus is vital before proceeding with UKA. If advanced osteoarthritic involvement and/or a compromised meniscus are discovered in the contralateral compartment, the previously planned UKA may be abandoned in favor of TKA, which is the preferred treatment option for advanced stages of knee OA. Thus, combining arthroscopy with UKA allows patients who are not appropriate candidates for UKA to be identified and excluded, thereby reducing the potential failure rate of UKA.[61]

The minimally invasive surgical approach must be differentiated from the mini-incision approach used by some surgeons. A mini incision is merely a small hole that may result in significant distortion of soft tissues, whereas the minimally invasive surgical technique preserves bone and the functioning of soft tissues. The advantages of the minimally invasive approach include a reduction in postoperative morbidity and pain, a decrease in rehabilitation time, and the ability to conduct the procedure on a same-day or short-stay basis.[14,17,39,42,44] In contrast, traditional TKA and UKA surgical approaches involve dislocation of the patella, which destroys the suprapatellar pouch and subsequently requires extensive physical therapy to reverse the ensuing iatrogenic damage. Repicci combines the minimally invasive surgical approach with the use of a resurfacing UKA design, which is referred to as minimally invasive UKA, to offer the additional benefit of minimal bone resection.

Minimally invasive UKA is highly advantageous because it avoids disturbing knee physiology, interfering with lifestyle, and interfering with future treatment options. Excluding the latter benefit, other surgeons[42-44] have applied this minimally invasive approach to other UKA designs and have reported successful outcomes. Rather than the small incision, the preservation of soft tissues and the avoidance of patellar dislocation are almost certainly responsible for the diminished postoperative pain and decreased rehabilitation time associated with minimally invasive UKA.[19,44,61] When it is presented as an arthritic bypass option with morbidity similar to arthroscopic procedures, patients with unicompartmental OA consistently choose minimally invasive UKA instead of TKA, preferring to delay a potential TKA for 8 to 10 years.[39]

According to the serial replacement philosophy advocated by Repicci and Hartman,[61] performing minimally invasive UKA in early, nonadvanced cases of OA, before TKA use and as a supplement to TKA, addresses patient satisfaction and prosthetic longevity. UKA used in this application absorbs approximately 10 years of functional capacity so that if and when future TKA is required, the survivability of the entire knee prosthetic system is extended to a 20- to 30-year range. The fundamental objective of this approach is to decrease the likelihood that a complex revision procedure will be required in a patient's lifetime. In addition, minimally invasive UKA has the extra benefit of addressing patient satisfaction issues, such as low morbidity, rapid rehabilitation, and less interference with lifestyle.

When UKA is used as part of a serial prosthetic replacement system, the indications may be expanded to include use in younger, more active patients; approximately 40% of Repicci's patients who present with unicompartmental OA qualify as candidates for the procedure. From its inception, this program was not designed to significantly alter the established UKA survivorship in the 90% range at 10 years.[2,15,27,32,47,62] Because of the limitations of today's technology, such survivorship is acceptable to Repicci, who uses UKA as a restoration procedure that supplements future TKA. However, for orthopaedic surgeons who use UKA as another salvage procedure, strict selection criteria are recommended to obtain survivorship similar to that of TKA,[3,15,42,47,50] the current gold-standard salvage procedure. Under stringent selection criteria, such as those described by Kozinn and Scott,[63] an estimated 6% to 12% of patients are eligible for UKA.[19,21,64]

THE FUTURE OF UNICONDYLAR KNEE ARTHROPLASTY

Opportunities remain for continued improvement of UKA. Due to the available surface area on the femur and by combining rounding resurfacing with the use of a fin for additional strength, femoral fixation in UKA appears to be adequately addressed. However, because the surface area of the tibia is approximately one fourth that of the femur, tremendous forces are placed on the tibia, making the tibial component the weakest link of UKA designs. The most common causes of UKA failure are tibial loosening[15,17,22,28,62] and polyethylene wear,[3,15,17,20,23,28] with aseptic loosening often occurring secondary to polyethylene wear.[3] Under current FDA regulations, a minimum polyethylene thickness of 6 mm is required for implantation,[17] and some orthopaedic surgeons[15,17] have recommended 8 mm as the minimum polyethylene thickness that should be implanted. Because the amount of space available for implantation of a UKA is limited and because of concerns about polyethylene wear, surgeons are faced with a paradox that perhaps is best summarized by Engh and associates:[29] "An inherent weakness of all unicompartmental implants is the need to use a relatively thin implant or to sacrifice additional bone."

The use of a thin all-polyethylene tibial component is not a viable solution because it is unable to withstand the high pressures resulting from small contact areas,[3] as demonstrated by past UKA failures involving the use of 6-mm tibial components.[3,6,19,26-28] However, significant tibial bone resections are not an ideal alternative because they may lead to considerable bone loss at the time of future revision to TKA, thereby interfering with future revision surgery and increasing the complexity of the revision procedure.[22,38] The metal-backed tibial components that were introduced to facilitate fixation and reduce polyethylene wear[3,15] require greater tibial resections due to the increased thickness of the components,[15] as well as the use of even thinner polyethylene.[19] In addition, the use of metal-backed components has resulted in the additional problem of polyethylene wear-through and an increased amount of wear.[2,29] Because polyethylene wear is reduced in mobile bearing UKA designs,[3,25,45] their use may solve the polyethylene dilemma; however, because of the significant resections required for their implantation, mobile bearing UKA designs do not resolve the issue of bone loss at the time of future revision.

Design improvements focusing on creating larger surface areas for bone ingrowth and/or using materials that promote such ingrowth are possible areas of exploration to increase tibial component stability. To use polyethylene to its full advantage, thicknesses in excess of 6 mm must be used for UKA tibial components. As a result of the

desire to minimize bone resections and subsequent bone loss at the time of future revision, the end of the polyethylene era in UKA may be near. The negative issues associated with polyethylene use include chemical, aging, wear, and deformity factors. Alternative materials with better wear properties for thinner layers, such as biologics, metal-on-metal, and polyethylene variants, may prove to be the ultimate solution to the UKA paradox.

CONCLUSION

The renewed interest in UKA in the United States, on the part of both orthopaedic surgeons and patients, coincides not only with improvement in surgical technique and design but also with the introduction of minimally invasive UKA.[16,65] This approach is significantly different from the use of a mini incision and is highly advantageous because it does not interfere with physiology, lifestyle, and future treatment options.[14] Avoiding patellar dislocation and nonessential tissue dissection results in lower morbidity and rapid rehabilitation. Because minimally invasive UKA may be performed on an outpatient basis, with full independence achieved by 4 hours postoperatively, rapid rehabilitation, and return to activities of daily living, it addresses patient satisfaction issues regarding lifestyle. Pain is managed through preoperative patient education, controlled anesthesia, local anesthetic infiltration of all incised tissues during surgery, avoidance of narcotics, and the use of only oral pain medication.

As a result of these advantages, the minimally invasive surgical approach used with UKA is increasing in popularity. Orthopaedic surgeons have started using this technique in conjunction with various philosophies regarding UKA design and application.[42-44] One school of thought advocates the use of a minimally invasive approach with resection UKA, asserting that with stringent selection criteria and proper surgical skill, resection UKA is an alternative salvage option to TKA.[15] The use of jigs often is recommended to assist with the surgical technique. Another philosophy involves the combination of a minimally invasive approach with mobile bearing UKA. According to this perspective, with proper surgical experience aided by the use of instrumentation and under strict indications,[2,42,47,50] the advantages of mobile bearing UKA designs, including low polyethylene wear, are maximized,[45] and survivorship comparable to TKA may be achieved.[2,42,47,50]

Common features of these two philosophies are the

adherence to strict selection criteria and the application of UKA as an alternative salvage option to be used instead of TKA. In contrast, Repicci recognizes the current limitations of UKA and, hence, uses minimally invasive UKA as a restoration procedure, supplementary to TKA. According to this concept, the minimally invasive approach is used in conjunction with resurfacing UKA, which has the added benefit of using sclerotic bone and preserving the medial tibial buttress without resecting valuable bone stock. This application of UKA does not interfere with future treatment options and is capable of extending the spectrum of knee survivability by approximately 10 years. Unlike TKA and the other UKA applications, this approach does not sacrifice significant bone and, consequently, complicate future revision surgery. In addition, because this arthritic bypass approach addresses the pathology of unicompartmental OA, it is an acceptable and often preferable alternative to procedures such as arthroscopic débridement and high tibial osteotomy.[5-7,20,32,55]

The benefits of using a minimally invasive approach with UKA, including a reduction in postoperative morbidity, a reduction in postoperative pain, a decrease in rehabilitation time, and the ability to conduct the procedure on a same-day or short-stay basis, are well recognized.[14,17,19,39,42,44] However, the type of UKA design and corresponding selection philosophy that will be the most advantageous remain to be seen as UKA volume increases and additional mid- to long-term survivorship studies of the various UKA applications are reported.

UKA remains a work-in-progress with further potential for improvement. An added benefit of the recent resurgence in UKA is the anticipation that increased funding will be allocated toward future research and development. In the end, it must be stressed that the single factor affecting survivorship of all UKAs, regardless of design or use of a minimally invasive approach, is proper surgical technique. Therefore, it is critical that surgeons who choose to pursue UKA receive proper training to ensure the surgical expertise required to successfully perform UKA.

REFERENCES

1. Insall JN, Clarke HD: Historic development, classification, and characteristics of knee prostheses, in Insall JN, Scott WN (eds): *Surgery of the Knee*, ed 3. New York, NY, Churchill Livingstone, 2001, pp 1516-1522.
2. Marmor L: The modular knee. *Clin Orthop* 1973;94:242-248.
3. Murray DW, Goodfellow JW, O'Connor JJ: The Oxford medial unicompartmental arthroplasty: A ten-year survival study. *J Bone Joint Surg Br* 1998;80:983-989.
4. Marmor L: The Marmor knee replacement. *Orthop Clin North Am* 1982;13:55-64.
5. Broughton NS, Newman JH, Baily RA: Unicompartmental replacement and high tibial osteotomy for osteoarthritis of the knee: A comparative study after 5-10 years' follow-up. *J Bone Joint Surg Br* 1986;68:447-452.
6. Marmor L: Unicompartmental knee arthroplasty of the knee with a minimum ten-year follow-up period. *Clin Orthop* 1988;228:171-177.
7. Scott RD, Santore RF: Unicondylar unicompartmental replacement for osteoarthritis of the knee. *J Bone Joint Surg Am* 1981;63:536-544.
8. Insall J, Aglietti P: A five to seven-year follow-up of unicondylar arthroplasty. *J Bone Joint Surg Am* 1980;62:1329-1337.
9. Insall J, Walker P: Unicondylar knee replacement. *Clin Orthop* 1976;120:83-85.
10. Laskin RS: Unicompartmental tibiofemoral resurfacing arthroplasty. *J Bone Joint Surg Am* 1978;60:182-185.
11. Dennis DA, Clayton ML, O'Donnell S, Mack RP, Stringer EA: Posterior cruciate condylar total knee arthroplasty: Average 11-year follow-up evaluation. *Clin Orthop* 1992;281:168-176.
12. Ritter MA, Campbell E, Faris PM, Keating EM: Long-term survival analysis of the posterior cruciate condylar total knee arthroplasty: A 10-year evaluation. *J Arthroplasty* 1989;4:293-296.
13. Scuderi GR, Insall JN, Windsor RE, Moran MC: Survivorship of cemented knee replacements. *J Bone Joint Surg Br* 1989;71:798-803.
14. Repicci JA, Eberle RW: Minimally invasive surgical technique for unicondylar knee arthroplasty. *J South Orthop Assoc* 1999;8:20-27.
15. Berger RA, Nedeff DD, Barden RM, et al: Unicompartmental knee arthroplasty: Clinical experience at 6- to 10-year follow-up. *Clin Orthop* 1999;367:50-60.
16. Bourne RB: Reevaluating the unicondylar knee arthroplasty. *Orthopedics* 2001;24:885-886.
17. Deshmukh RV, Scott RD: Unicompartmental knee arthroplasty: Long-term results. *Clin Orthop* 2001;392:272-278.
18. Grelsamer RP, Cartier P: A unicompartmental knee replacement is not "half a total knee:" Five major differences. *Orthop Rev* 1992;21:1350-1356.
19. Laskin RS: Unicompartmental knee replacement: Some unanswered questions. *Clin Orthop* 2001;392:267-271.
20. McAuley JP, Engh GA, Ammeen DJ: Revision of failed unicompartmental knee arthroplasty. *Clin Orthop* 2001;392:279-282.

21. Sculco TP: Orthopaedic crossfire: Can we justify uni-condylar arthroplasty as a temporizing procedure? In opposition. *J Arthroplasty* 2002;17(suppl 1):56-58.

22. Barrett WP, Scott RD: Revision of failed unicondylar unicompartmental knee arthroplasty. *J Bone Joint Surg Am* 1987;69:1328-1335.

23. Bohm I, Landsiedl F: Revision surgery after failed unicompartmental knee arthroplasty: A study of 35 cases. *J Arthroplasty* 2000;15:982-989.

24. Levine WN, Ozuna RM, Scott RD, Thornhill TS: Conversion of failed modern unicompartmental arthroplasty to total knee arthroplasty. *J Arthroplasty* 1996;11:797-801.

25. Lindstrand A, Stenstrom A, Ryd L, Toksvig-Larsen S: The introduction period of unicompartmental knee arthroplasty is critical: A clinical, clinical multicentered, and radiostereometric study of 251 Duracon unicompartmental knee arthroplasties. *J Arthroplasty* 2000;15:608-616.

26. Marmor L: Results of single compartment arthroplasty with acrylic cement fixation: A minimum follow-up of two years. *Clin Orthop* 1977;122:181-188.

27. Cartier P, Sanouiller JL, Grelsamer RP: Unicompartmental knee arthroplasty surgery: 10-year minimum follow-up period. *J Arthroplasty* 1996;11:782-788.

28. Engh GA, McAuley JP: Unicondylar arthroplasty: an option for high-deman patients with gonarthrosis. *Instr Course Lect* 1999;48:143-148.

29. Engh GA, Dwyer KA, Hanes CK: Polyethylene wear of metal-backed tibial components in total and unicompartmental knee prostheses. *J Bone Joint Surg Br* 1992;74:9-17.

30. Lindstrand A, Stenstrom A, Lewold S: Multicenter study of unicompartmental knee revision: PCA, Marmor, and St. Georg compared in 3,777 cases of arthrosis. *Acta Orthop Scand* 1992;63:256-259.

31. Grelsamer RP: Unicompartmental osteoarthrosis of the knee. *J Bone Joint Surg Am* 1995;77:278-292.

32. Squire MW, Callaghan JJ, Goetz DD, Sullivan PM, Johnston RC: Unicompartmental knee replacement: A minimum 15 year follow-up study. *Clin Orthop* 1999;367:61-72.

33. Bert JM: Universal intramedullary instrumentation for unicompartmental total knee arthroplasty. *Clin Orthop* 1991;271:79-87.

34. Knutson K, Lewold S, Robertsson O, Lidgren L: The Swedish knee arthroplasty register: A nation-wide study of 30,003 knees 1976-1992. *Acta Orthop Scand* 1994;65:375-386.

35. Lewold S, Knutson K, Lidgren L: Reduced failure rate in knee prosthetic surgery with improved implantation technique. *Clin Orthop* 1993;287:94-97.

36. Ahlback S: Osteoarthrosis of the knee: A radiographic investigation. *Acta Radiol Diagn (Stockholm)* 1968;277(suppl):7-72.

37. Hernborg JS, Nilsson BE: The natural course of untreated osteoarthritis of the knee. *Clin Orthop* 1977;123:130-137.

38. Padgett DE, Stern SH, Insall JN: Revision total knee arthroplasty for failed unicompartmental replacement. *J Bone Joint Surg Am* 1991;73:186-190.

39. Romanowski MR, Repicci JA: Minimally invasive unicondylar arthroplasty: Eight-year follow-up. *J Knee Surg* 2002;15:17-22.

40. Weale AE, Halabi OA, Jones PW, White SH: Perceptions of outcomes after unicompartmental and total knee replacements. *Clin Orthop* 2001;382:143-153.

41. Knutson K, Lewold S, Lidgren L: Outcome of revision for failed unicompartmental knee arthroplasty for arthrosis. Presented as a Poster Exhibit at the American Academy of Orthopaedic Surgeons meeting, Washington, 1992.

42. Murray DW: Unicompartmental knee replacement: now or never? *Orthopedics* 2000;23:979-980.

43. Price A, Webb J, Topf H, Dodd C, Goodfellow J, Murray D: Abstract: Oxford unicompartmental knee replacement with a minimally invasive technique. *J Bone Joint Surg Br* 2000;82(suppl 1):24.

44. Price AJ, Webb J, Topf H, Dodd CA, Goodfellow JW, Murray DW: Rapid recovery after oxford unicompartmental arthroplasty through a short incision. *J Arthroplasty* 2001;16:970-976.

45. Psychoyios V, Crawford RW, O'Connor JJ, Murray DW: Wear of congruent meniscal bearings in unicompartmental knee arthroplasty: A retrieval study of 16 specimens. *J Bone Joint Surg Br* 1998;80:976-982.

46. Lewold S, Goodman S, Knutson K, Robertsson O, Lidgren L: Oxford meniscal bearing knee versus the Marmor knee in unicompartmental arthroplasty for arthrosis: A Swedish multicenter survival study. *J Arthroplasty* 1995;10:722-731.

47. Svard UC, Price AJ: Oxford medial unicompartmental knee arthroplasty: A survival analysis of an independent series. *J Bone Joint Surg Br* 2001;83:191-194.

48. Gunther T, Murray DW, Miller R, et al: Lateral unicompartmental arthroplasty with the Oxford meniscal knee. *Knee* 1996;3:33-39.

49. Robertsson O, Knutson K, Lewold S, Lidgren L: The routine of surgical management reduces failure after unicompartmental knee arthroplasty. *J Bone Joint Surg Br* 2001;83:45-49.

50. Vorlat P, Verdonk R, Schauvlieghe H: The Oxford unicompartmental knee prosthesis: A 5-year follow-up. *Knee Surg Sports Traumatol Arthrosc* 2000;8:154-158.

51. Bartley RE, Stulberg SD, Robb WJ III, Sweeney HJ: Polyethylene wear in unicompartmental knee arthroplasty. *Clin Orthop* 1994;299:18-24.

52. Baumgaertner MR, Cannon WD Jr, Vittori JM, Schmidt ES, Maurer RC: Arthroscopic debridement of the arthritic knee. *Clin Orthop* 1990;253:197-202.

53. Gibson JN, White MD, Chapman VM, Strachan RK: Arthroscopic lavage and debridement for osteoarthritis of the knee. *J Bone Joint Surg Br* 1992;74:534-537.

54. Insall JN, Joseph DM, Msika C: High tibial osteotomy for varus gonarthrosis: A long-term follow-up study. *J Bone Joint Surg Am* 1984;66:1040-1048.

55. Karpman RR, Volz RG: Osteotomy versus unicompartmental prosthetic replacement in the treatment of unicompartmental arthritis of the knee. *Orthopedics* 1982;5:989-991.

56. Matthews LS, Goldstein SA, Malvitz TA, Katz BP, Kaufer H: Proximal tibial osteotomy: Factors that influence the duration of satisfactory function. *Clin Orthop* 1988;229:193-200.

57. Moseley JB, O'Malley K, Petersen NJ, et al: A controlled trial of arthroscopic surgery for osteoarthritis of the knee. *N Engl J Med* 2002;347:81-88.

58. Kettlekamp DB, Jacobs AW: Tibiofemoral contact area: Determination and implications. *J Bone Joint Surg Am* 1972;54:349-356.

59. Kuster MA, Wood GA, Stachowiak GW, Gachter A: Joint load considerations in total knee replacement. *J Bone Joint Surg Br* 1997;79:109-113.

60. Walker PS, Erkman MJ: The role of the menisci in force transmission across the knee. *Clin Orthop* 1975;109:184-192.

61. Repicci JA, Hartman JF: Minimally invasive unicondylar knee arthroplasty for the treatment of unicompartmental osteoarthritis: An out-patient arthritic bypass procedure. *Orthop Clin North Am.* in press.

62. Heck DA, Marmor L, Gibson A, Rougraff BT: Unicompartmental knee arthroplasty: A multicenter investigation with long-term follow-up evaluation. *Clin Orthop* 1993;286:154-159.

63. Kozinn SC, Scott R: Unicondylar knee arthroplasty. *J Bone Joint Surg Am* 1989;71:145-150.

64. Stern SH, Becker MW, Insall JN: Unicondylar knee arthroplasty: An evaluation of selection criteria. *Clin Orthop* 1993;286:143-148.

65. Engh GA: Orthopaedic crossfire: Can we justify unicondylar arthroplasty as a temporizing procedure? In the affirmative. *J Arthroplasty* 2002;17(suppl 4):54-55.